Praise for Terry and *Discovering*

D1489236

"Terry Lemerond is a maverick. He is a legend in his o̶ɴ̶...̶ld of evidence-based natural medicine. His passion for knowledge and his strong, heartfelt desire to share it has made the world a much better place. I am honored to not only know this man, but to have had the chance to work with him and learn from him."

—**Holly Lucille, ND, RN**, nationally recognized educator, practitioner, author, natural products consultant, and television and radio host

"Have you been failed by the medical profession? Help is on the way! After 40 years as a physician, and having reviewed tens of thousands of studies, I have found that there is a simple way to learn what natural treatments will be future superstars. Simply see what Terry Lemerond is talking about today!"

—**Jacob Teitelbaum, MD**, Director of the Fatigue and Fibromyalgia Practitioners Network, practitioner, researcher, and expert in chronic pain. Author of multiple best-selling books including *Fatigued to Fantastic*. Lead author of the SHINE protocol for Chronic Fatigue Syndrome and Fibromyalgia

"Terry Lemerond is a walking encyclopedia when it comes to natural cures, botanicals, and nutraceuticals. The formulator of over 400 products, he knows as much about what works and what doesn't as anyone I've ever met. He's one of a handful of people in the natural products industry who really deserves the designation 'icon.' I've learned a ton from Terry—read this book and you'll see why!"

—**Jonny Bowden, PhD, CNS**, best-selling author, radio host, speaker, and national media health expert on weight loss, nutrition, and health with six national certifications in personal training and exercise

"Terry has been a pioneer for natural health products for close to fifty years, and through these years he has found countless, life-changing ingredients that really have made a tremendous impact on people's health. I have never met anyone during my tenure in the natural health industry with such vision for finding the best quality and unique ingredients around the world. Not only has Terry contributed incredible products and been the first to introduce some of these ingredients to North America, he has inspired so many with his kindness, passion, dedication, and love for people and natural health. He speaks from a place of personal experience, and through this his love for what he does shines brightly. I am blessed to know Terry both personally and professionally, and it is an honor to call him my friend."

—**Karlene Karst, RD**, best-selling author, and recognized authority on the role of natural food and wholesome ingredients in nutrition, author, and founder of Sea-licious

"Due to my academic research, I have had the privilege of getting to meet some of the leading authorities in the world on the medicinal benefits of botanicals and phytochemicals. However, I must say Terry is, without a question, one of the most well-versed and knowledgeable individuals I have ever had the privilege and honor of getting to know. His breadth of understanding on a large number of plants and herbs amazes me, but what is more fascinating is his depth of scientific knowledge on these products—which is truly remarkable and exceptional. All of this is fueled by Terry's unparalleled passion for learning and educating consumers on the health benefits of nature's cures."

—**Ajay Goel, PhD**, Professor and the Director of Translational Genomics and Oncology, and the Director of the Center for Gastrointestinal Research at the Baylor Scott & White Research Institute, Baylor University Medical Center in Dallas, TX., member of American Cancer Association for Research and the American Gastroenterology Association, and one of the top scientists in the world investigating botanical interventions.

"From the viewpoint of an editor of scientific journals on phytomedicine and phytotherapy research, this guide for the novice consumer of dietary supplements is surprisingly different from many handbooks on herbal medicines. This book was written by a pioneer in natural health products, a walking encyclopedia, and a revolutionary thinker. I want to emphasize that this evidence based information is a summary of selected medicinal plants and supplements, covering all of the most essential health conditions that is valuable for a consumer. The consumer should read this book."

—**Alexander Panossian PhD, Dr.Sc.**, has advanced research degrees in bioorganic chemistry and specializes in the study of adaptogenic herbs. He has authored or co-authored over 170 scientific publications. Dr. Panossian is a past Editor-in-Chief of *Phytomedicine*.

"Terry Lemerond is the reason I was drawn into the world of natural health. His passion is contagious and his magnificent knowledge of natural supplements set me on the road to becoming an integrative medicine practitioner and professional lecturer. I am proud to call him my teacher, my mentor, and my friend. His book is a perfect doorway into the world of clinically validated, highly effective natural interventions for some of the most serious health problems facing people today. If you have health questions, your answers begin in this book."

—**Cheryl Myers, RN, BA**, is an integrative health care professional, research liaison, author, lecturer, and natural products expert. Her blogs and columns can be found in *Taste for Life, MindBodyGreen,* and *Vitamin Retailer*.

Discovering Your Best Health

TERRY LEMEROND

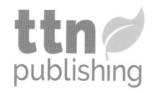

ttn
publishing

ISBN: 978-1-952507-31-1

Editor: Kim Erickson
Interior: Gary A. Rosenberg • www.thebookcouple.com

Printed in the United States of America

10   9   8   7   6   5   4   3   2   1

Contents

OTHER BOOKS BY TERRY LEMEROND

50+ Natural Health Secrets Proven to Change Your Life!

Seven Keys to Unlimited Personal Achievement

Seven Keys to Vibrant Health

Preface

Life expectancy in the U.S. is at an all-time high. And for many people, the possibility of living a longer life holds the promise of more postretirement years free from the grind of work and responsibilities. Yet the dream of a retirement filled with more time to travel the world, more time to enjoy long neglected hobbies, and more time to spend with family and friends could be just that—a dream. Why? Because if you're living a typical American lifestyle, you may not be healthy enough to relish those golden years.

• • • • • • • • • •

Don't believe me? Just look at the numbers. According to the Centers for Disease Control and Prevention (CDC), 6 in 10 Americans are living with at least one chronic disease. Among those who are 60 years old or older, at least 80 percent have one chronic illness and 50 percent are living with two. What's even more surprising is that nearly 30 million Americans are living with five or more chronic conditions!

A disease is considered chronic when it lasts for at least a year and requires ongoing medical treatment or medication. These conditions may limit the activities you can participate in and likely have a negative impact on your quality of life. The most common chronic illnesses include:

✦ Alzheimer's disease or some other form of dementia

✦ Arthritis

✦ Cancer

✦ Chronic obstructive pulmonary disease (COPD)

✦ Coronary artery disease

✦ Depression

✦ Heart failure

✦ High blood pressure (hypertension)

✦ Kidney disease

✦ Obesity

✦ Osteoporosis

✦ Type 2 diabetes

Dealing with even one of these diseases, much less two or more, can upend your lifestyle, zap your energy, and drain your wallet. And yet, conventional medical experts would have you believe that many of these conditions and their symptoms, such as joint pain, memory loss, or weight gain, are simply a normal part of aging. For the conditions they can't shove into the "aging" category, these experts are happy to prescribe a litany of pharmaceutical drugs to help manage your symptoms.

It's this pill-popping, quick-fix approach that's created a health crisis in America. Nowhere in the conventional medical system are doctors taught to practice preventive care or to foster optimal health using the time-honored tools of diet, exercise, dietary supplements, mind-body strategies, or other health-promoting therapies. In fact, medical students only receive an average of 23.9 hours of nutritional instruction during their training. And only 40 medical schools require the minimum 25 hours of nutrition education recommended by the National Academy of Sciences.

Instead, modern Western medicine is centered around a narrow scientific model that relies on animal and human studies which are often faulty in their design and frequently paid for by the pharmaceutical industry. These studies also foster the belief that the human body is a complex machine made up of individual parts that can be treated independently rather than as an integrated whole. By looking at only one part of the anatomy, physicians all too easily view the patient as a test subject instead of an equal partner in the healing process. How patients are feeling, their environment, or their daily habits are often discounted. Instead, everyone who experiences the same symptoms or disease gets treated with the same protocol. It's a system that's rigged to keep paying patients alive but not necessarily healthy.

This may leave you wondering, what's the point of living a long life if it's not a healthy one? But here's the good news: declining health isn't inevitable. There are numerous things you can do to live a long and healthy life. *You* have the power to take charge of your health and your happiness.

I know what you're thinking, and it's true—there are hundreds of books on the market offering conflicting advice on diet, exercise, supplementation, sleep, and so much more. So why am I adding to the mix? Because people need a simple road map based on credible science to help them achieve their best health—no gimmicks, no celebrities, no trendy new tricks that supposedly provide instant results. Just health strategies that truly work. What's more, the information you'll find in the following chapters isn't purely academic, and it doesn't simply regurgitate conventional health advice. The strategies here are based on cutting-edge science and my own personal experience gained over 50 years in the natural health industry. Best of all, the healthy tips and habits you'll learn about actually work. I know because these are habits I practice every day.

I discovered the power of healthy living and supplementation firsthand during my younger years. Like many Americans, I grew up consuming junk food, candy, and soft drinks at every opportunity. By the time I celebrated my 20th birthday, I weighed more than 250 pounds. Now, that would have been fine if I had been 6'5" tall—but because I measured just 5'6", I was wider than I was high! But my problems weren't just confined to my weight. Because I wasn't giving my body or my brain the nutrients they needed, I battled severe hypoglycemia and severe depression. I was extremely unhappy. As a result, I was also obnoxious, belligerent, and very angry.

My wake-up call came when a respected priest at the Catholic school I attended took me under his wing and told me in no uncertain terms that if I continued down the path I was on, I would certainly land in jail. I got the message. So, instead of heading off to college, I joined the Marines in hopes of getting my life together. What I got was so much more.

While stationed at Camp Pendleton I joined the weight-lifting team and met Captain Ed Vito, who took on the role of my mentor. He suggested ways that I could improve my diet, starting with fruits, vegetables, whole grains, and some foods I had never even heard of. Over time, I lost weight and put on muscle, looking better than I ever had. Captain Vito also introduced me to a little health-food store

in Oceanside, California. Coming from Green Bay, Wisconsin, in the late 1950s, the concept of a health-food store was new to me, but I was instantly transfixed by the rows of supplements that lined the store's shelves. It was the final piece of the puzzle in my journey toward good mental and physical health.

By the time I left the Marine Corps, I was a changed man. I was physically fit, my blood sugar levels had stabilized, and the cloud of depression had lifted. For the first time in my life, I was healthy and happy.

During the interim years, I've devoted my life to empowering others by helping them realize their own health potential. I've owned health-food stores, launched two successful dietary-supplement companies, hosted a radio show, and introduced several important nutrients to consumers in the U.S., including milk thistle, ginkgo biloba, deglycyrrhizinated licorice (DGL), and glucosamine sulfate. But the most important and rewarding thing I do when I wake up every morning is sharing the knowledge I've gained over the years about the many (often simple) ways to optimize people's health and well-being.

If knowledge is power, then you hold the power of good health in your hands.

Introduction

What does it mean to be healthy? Most people—including a surprising number of doctors—believe that if you aren't sick, you're healthy. While this simplistic viewpoint might be comforting to some, the absence of disease doesn't necessarily mean that you're healthy. The truth is, your environment and daily habits can, over time, either enhance your health or undermine it.

• • • • • • • • • •

And that means *you* are largely in control of your own health, for better or for worse.

Now don't get me wrong. I'm not insinuating that you don't need a doctor or conventional medical care. I'm all for conventional medicine when an accident or an emergency occurs. But when it comes to optimizing your health, far too many doctors are clueless. They specialize in evaluating symptoms, dispensing drugs, and performing surgery. Instead of practicing health care, what most conventional doctors actually practice is sick care. And, although that can play an important role

in medicine, it's so much better to prevent disease in the first place. And that means educating and empowering people to take the actions needed to foster their best health. And one of the smartest places to start is with those habits they practice day in and day out.

How much do your daily choices impact your health? According to British researchers who followed 4,886 people for more than 20 years, they matter a lot. During their study, which appeared in the journal *Archives of Internal Medicine,* the researchers found that people who are sedentary, eat a nutrient-poor diet filled with ultra-processed foods, smoke, and frequently overindulge in alcohol are three times more likely to die of some form of cardiovascular disease and nearly four times more likely to die of cancer. What's more, people who practice all four of these unhealthy habits have a biological age that's 12 years older than their healthy counterparts!

On the flip side, another large study—this one conducted by Harvard investigators—found that people who adopted healthier habits had a significantly lower risk of dying of heart disease, cancer, or other chronic illness. This study looked at the long-term effects of five healthy habits among more than 78,000 women and 44,000 men. The habits included eating a healthy diet, not smoking, getting at least three and a half hours of moderate to vigorous exercise each week, drinking only moderate amounts of alcohol, and maintaining a healthy weight. During the 34-year follow-up, the Harvard team noted that the women who didn't practice any of these habits lived, on average, to the age of 79, whereas the men only made it to 75. But the women who embraced all five healthy habits lived to see their 93rd birthday. The men also lived longer, with an average life expectancy of nearly 88 years old. And those extra years were healthy, happy, and active ones.

These studies clearly show that the habits you practice every single day matter. But, you might be wondering, what about the genes you inherited? Don't they boost your odds of developing the same diseases your parents or grandparents had? I'll let you in on a little secret: your genes are not your destiny.

How Your Lifestyle Affects Your Genes . . .

Anyone who's taken basic high school biology knows that your DNA makes you who you are. It's that unique double helix–shaped coding that exists deep within your cells that's responsible for the color of your eyes and hair, your height, and the diseases you may be more prone to develop. Your personal DNA and the clues it may hold

regarding future disease is why, when you go in for a routine physical, your doctor asks about your family history. For instance, if your mother suffered from atherosclerosis and your father was treated for skin cancer, you may be at a higher risk of developing these conditions because of the genes you inherited from them.

Your DNA is a code that stores biological data in your genes. First identified by Swiss physiological chemist Friedrich Miescher in 1869, the twisted ladder-like structure we now know as DNA was introduced by two University of Cambridge scientists, Francis Crick and James Watson, in 1953. Their discoveries led to the Human Genome Project, an international research program whose goal was to identify and map all of the genes that make humans, well...human.

Your genetic code is as individual as you are. But your DNA isn't made up of static microscopic structures that dictate your future health. Instead, it's a dynamic and adaptable set of molecules that form your own personal genome—a detailed blueprint of instructions for your body. Your genes tell your body when to make certain proteins. These proteins don't just determine the color of your eyes; they also power your muscles, govern how your immune cells react to invading pathogens, and so much more.

But even though your genes control much of your physiology, they can also be controlled by your environment and your actions. This field of study, known as epigenetics, increasingly shows how external factors like your diet and level of physical activity, the chemicals you encounter, or the things you experience can turn genes on or off, influencing how they function.

Here's just one example: in a Swedish study, researchers at Lund University found that people who ate diets high in ultra-processed carbohydrates experienced an overexpression of genes associated with cardiovascular disease. In another study, which was presented at the 2019 meeting of the European and International Congress on Obesity, Spanish researchers reported that people eating diets high in ultra-processed foods weren't just overweight or obese; they also had a significantly higher biological age. While your chronological age is simply a record of the number of years you've been alive, your biological age reflects your inner age. Your biological age takes into account your lifestyle and the many ways your everyday habits impact how your genes are expressed. This means that, although you might be 50 years old chronologically, if you live an unhealthy lifestyle, your biological age might be 62. Fortunately, the reverse is also true. If you eat a healthy diet, exercise, get plenty of good-quality sleep, and avoid unhealthy habits like smoking, your biological age could be far younger than your chronological age.

Your long-term habits don't just have the ability to turn your genes off and on; they can also shorten your telomeres. Not familiar with telomeres or the role they play in epigenetics? You're not alone! In fact, most scientists were pretty clueless until three researchers won the Nobel Prize in Physiology or Medicine in 2009 after discovering that telomeres play a key role in protecting DNA.

Here's how it works: Your telomeres are protective caps found on the ends of your chromosomes, kind of like the plastic caps on the ends of your shoelaces. Because they safeguard the DNA inside your chromosomes, they can keep your cells from aging. But if your telomeres become shorter, your cells age faster than they normally would. And that was exactly what the Spanish researchers discovered when they dug deeper into their findings. It turns out that those participants who consumed large amounts of sugar-sweetened beverages, alcohol, and ultra-processed foods high in unhealthy fats and sugar had shorter telomeres—and that's what led to an older biological age.

. . . And Your Gut

Your genes aren't the only things affected by your lifestyle. The bacteria in your gut can also fall victim to an unhealthy lifestyle. Or to be more specific, your bacteria's genes.

Your body is home to some 100 trillion microorganisms, including bacteria, viruses, parasites, and fungi. Most of these microbes live in your large intestine, often simply referred to as your gut. This collection of microbes is known in scientific circles as your microbiota, and their health and well-being are dependent on something called the microbiome. And here's where things get really interesting: Your microbiome is actually the combined genetic material of all the microorganisms that live in and on your body. And surprisingly, those microbes contain 3.3 million genes compared to just 23,000 human genes. If you did the math, out of the 100 trillion cells that make up your body, only about 1 in 10 is actually human!

Your gut alone contains more than 500 different strains of bacteria—some good and some bad. Your good bacteria works hard to protect against the bad bugs that can make you sick. They do this by producing organic compounds such as lactic acid, hydrogen peroxide, and acetic acid. These compounds boost the acidity in your intestinal tract, preventing the harmful microbes from reproducing. The beneficial bacteria in your gut also produces a natural antibiotic, called bacteriocin, that kills off harmful microbes and works with your immune system to increase the number of disease-fighting cells that could prevent sickness.

In a perfect world, your good and bad bacteria would live in harmony. In the real world, however, this balance is often out of whack—largely because of your lifestyle choices. It turns out that, just like the DNA that makes you who you are can be impacted by your lifestyle choices, your bacteria's DNA is also subject to epigenetic changes. As a result, your microbiome can be affected by what you eat, the amount of exercise and sleep you get, the amount of stress you're under, and even what you touch in your environment. And that can have far-reaching effects on your overall health.

As the scientific community began to connect the dots on the role the microbiome plays in human health, they also began looking for possible links between the state of the microbiome and a variety of diseases. What they found was truly astounding.

In recent years, studies have linked an unhealthy microbiome to a number of chronic conditions, including anxiety, autoimmune problems, cancer, diabetes, heart disease, inflammatory bowel disease, obesity, and even vision loss. One study found that people with coronary artery disease and heart failure have one thing in common—a decrease in the production of two protective compounds in the gut, butyrate and trimethylamine N-oxide. Since these two important compounds are involved in regulating the immune system's inflammatory response and preventing atherosclerosis, it's easy to see how an unbalanced microbiome—technically called dysbiosis—can contribute to several forms of heart disease, such as high blood pressure and coronary artery disease.

Dysbiosis also contributes to a greater risk of type 2 diabetes. Some studies have found that a bacterial imbalance weakens the intestinal barrier and triggers chronic low-grade inflammation in people dealing with obesity and type 2 diabetes. If you don't repair the microbiota with diet, exercise, and stress management, this increase in inflammation can lead to even more insulin resistance, creating a vicious cycle.

Maybe the most surprising connection is how your microbiome affects your brain—or more specifically, how it affects your odds of developing Alzheimer's disease. Still incurable, Alzheimer's and other types of dementia directly affect six million Americans. That translates to about one in every three seniors. By 2050, the Alzheimer's Association projects that 13 million people will be living with the disease. Although Alzheimer's is an extremely complex disease and science is still uncovering the condition's many twists and turns, there is some progress. A team of European scientists recently made the connection between an imbalance in the gut microbiome and the development of amyloid plaque in the brain—a hallmark of Alzheimer's. During the study, which appeared in the *Journal of Alzheimer's Disease,* the scientists concluded that proteins produced by certain strains of beneficial gut bacteria might likely change the way the immune system and the nervous system interact to trigger the disease. This offers the hope of creating new ways to prevent Alzheimer's and other types of neurodegenerative diseases.

But even though the mechanisms that lead to disease might seem complicated, the fix is simple. And you don't even need to wait for some new miracle pill to treat the things that ail you. You already have everything you need right here in this book to balance your microbiome and dial in your epigenetic potential. This not only helps protect against a litany of chronic conditions; it can also help you optimize your health so you can enjoy a long and vibrant life.

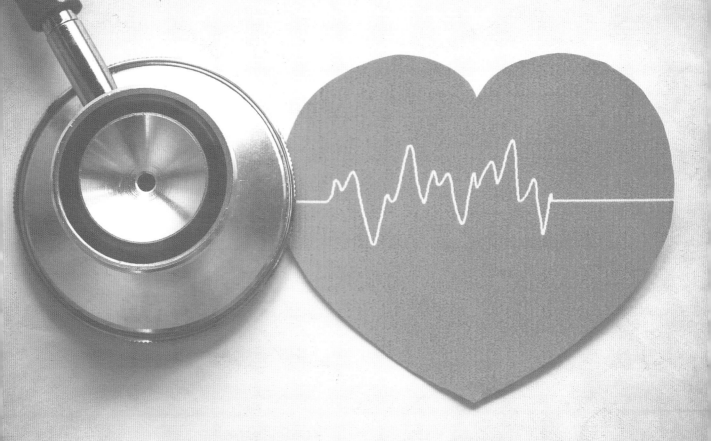

SECTION ONE

FOOD FIRST

CHAPTER 1

You Really Are What You Eat

What did you eat today? Perhaps you started your day with coffee and a pastry, then grabbed a burger and fries that you washed down with a sugary soda for lunch. By the end of the day, you're too tired to cook so you order takeout for dinner before settling into your favorite chair for a night's worth of TV and microwave popcorn. This is the way millions of Americans eat every day. And I get it—it's easy and it's tasty. But it's also killing you.

· · · · · · · · · · ·

Just look at the statistics. The percentage of people who are overweight in the U.S. has reached astronomical numbers. According to the Harvard T.H. Chan School of Public Health, 71.6 percent of adults over the age of 20 are now considered to be overweight. Of those, 42.4 percent are obese—up from 30.5 percent in 2000. This trend costs the medical system a whopping $200 billion each year. On a more personal level, obesity can cost nearly $5,000 more in healthcare costs annually for women and $2,600 for men.

But if you're overweight, the cost to your health can be considerably higher than the cost to your pocketbook. Numerous studies show a distinct link between obesity and a litany of chronic conditions, including cancer, chronic pain, coronary artery disease, depression and anxiety, gall bladder disease, joint problems, high blood pressure, nonalcoholic fatty liver disease, sleep apnea, stroke, type 2 diabetes, unhealthy cholesterol and triglyceride levels, not to mention greater odds of dying prematurely. Even if you don't develop any of these conditions, you'll likely have difficulty performing everyday tasks like climbing stairs or even just bending over to tie your shoes. Either way, obesity often results in a lower overall quality of life.

Let's take a deeper dive into what makes so many of the foods we eat so unhealthy and how they're fueling disease (and maybe even an early demise).

Some studies estimate that 300,000 people die of obesity in the U.S. every year.

Is Your Diet SAD?

It's true. America really is the land of plenty. Plenty of ultra-processed foods and fast-food restaurants, that is. And all this plenty is making us sick.

These unhealthy foods increasingly make up the Standard American Diet, a diet with the fitting acronym SAD. What makes this diet so sad? Instead of providing nutrient-rich fruits and vegetables, high-quality protein, and healthy fats that foster good health, the food industry transforms otherwise good-for-you ingredients into unrecognizable morsels packed with salt, refined sugar, cheap pro-inflammatory fats, chemical preservatives, and artificial flavors and colors. These foods are not only short on nutrients, but they're long on ingredients shown to trigger chronic inflammation, disrupt your microbiome, and upend the way your genes function. This can, over time, open the door to weight gain, disease, and quite possibly premature death.

Why would food companies deliberately create such unhealthy foods? Just follow the money. If you've ever seen the iconic 1987 movie Wall Street, you may remember Gordon Gekko's famous line "greed is good." And it's this greed that's at the root of the food industry's practices. To maximize their profits, ultra-processed-food giants like General Mills, Kraft, Nestlé, and Tyson Foods employ thousands of food scientists to create cheap, ready-to-eat foods that taste good and can sit in warehouses or on store shelves for months or even years. Accomplishing this typically requires plentiful low-cost ingredients such as refined sugars, white flour, and processed vegetable fats high in calories and low in nutrients. Another frequent addition? Chemical additives like MSG that enhance flavor, and sketchy preservatives like butylated hydroxyanisole (BHA) and butylated hydroxytoluene (BHT) that prevent rancidity. What's missing? Fiber, minerals, vitamins, and other nutrients essential for good health.

While some ultra-processed foods are obvious—think chicken nuggets, artificially flavored chips, and sodas—others may be a little harder to spot. Consider a bottle of Italian salad dressing. On its face you might think it contains oil, vinegar, and a handful of herbs. But if you take a look at the ingredient label, you'll likely discover that your seemingly benign salad dressing not only contains cheap canola oil, which triggers inflammation; it also harbors a variety of sugars and a laundry list of tongue-twisting preservatives, flavors, and colors.

Industrial food scientists have also made moves on the health-food market. Although many large natural-food markets carry an array of unhealthy chips, cookies, and other highly processed junk foods (often under the guise of organic or non-GMO), I believe that plant-based meat substitutes like Beyond Meat or Impossible "meats" are the absolute worst ultra-processed foods sold under the "health food" banner. Just take a look at the ingredients found in many of these faux meats, along with their potential health risks:

INGREDIENT	HEALTH EFFECTS
Artificial colors	Blue 1, Red 40, Yellow 5, and Yellow 6 are made from petroleum, and they can cause allergic reactions and disrupt the immune system. Numerous studies have also found that these dyes cause hyperactivity in children.
Artificial flavors	There are over 3,000 different chemicals allowed to be used as artificial flavors for foods in the U.S. These ingredients can trigger allergic reactions, dysbiosis, fatigue, headache, and hyperactivity. Some have been shown to be carcinogenic.
Autolyzed yeast extract	High in salt, some yeast extracts can cause headaches.
Bleached wheat flour	Bleaching flour requires the use of up to 20 dubious chemicals, such as benzoyl peroxide and chlorine gas, which remain in the finished product in trace amounts. The process also breaks down any nutrients naturally found in wheat.
Canola oil	This ubiquitous oil is created using hexane, a solvent that is a known neurotoxin suspected of damaging reproductive and fetal health. Nearly all canola oil is derived from genetically modified rapeseed plants.
Caramel color	Some types of caramel color produce carcinogenic byproducts that can remain in the finished product.
Carrageenan	Used as a thickener, carrageenan can cause intestinal inflammation, bloating, and irritable bowel syndrome. It may also increase the risk of colon cancer.
Corn oil	Corn oil is heavily processed using hexane, a known human neurotoxin that may damage reproductive and fetal health. Most corn grown in the U.S. is genetically modified.
Corn syrup solids	A corn-based sweetener high in fructose that may contribute to heart disease and obesity, this additive is also listed on food labels as high-fructose corn syrup (HFCS).
Hydrolyzed vegetable protein	Made from corn, soy, or wheat that is boiled in hydrochloric acid and neutralized with sodium hydroxide—a process that creates small amounts of MSG.
Hydrolyzed wheat gluten	A heavily processed additive used to make ingredients stick together, it's unsuitable for those with celiac disease or a gluten sensitivity.
Maltodextrin	This highly processed thickener can cause spikes in blood sugar, as well as give harmful bacteria like *salmonella* and *E. coli* a better chance at surviving in the digestive tract.

INGREDIENT	HEALTH EFFECTS
Methylcellulose	This cheap additive adds bulk to and improves the texture of products without adding any nutritional benefits.
Modified food starch	Modified food starch is treated with chemicals, including chlorine, hydrogen peroxide, potassium permanganate, sodium hypochlorite, and acids, to improve its texture at higher temperatures. It is used to add bulk to and improve the texture of processed foods.
Natural flavors	Often the sign of a low-quality food, these highly processed flavors aren't typically derived from the food they are mimicking.
Propylene glycol	This food additive is also used to make antifreeze. While generally considered safe, it can be toxic if ingested in large amounts.
Sodium phosphate	This preservative is a source of excess dietary phosphorus that can lead to cardiovascular and kidney problems. The body absorbs roughly twice as much phosphorus from additives as it does from natural sources.
Sodium tripolyphosphate	This synthetic preservative is a source of excess dietary phosphorous that can cause cardiovascular and kidney problems. According to the National Institute for Occupational Safety and Health, sodium tripolyphosphate is a suspected neurotoxin that can cause digestive distress.
Soy lecithin	Extracted from soybeans using hexane, a known neurotoxin that may damage reproductive and fetal health.
Soy protein	Soy protein isolates and concentrates are made by separating soy proteins from fats using hexane. Most soy in foods sold in the U.S. is genetically modified.
Sugar	Added sugars increase the risk of Alzheimer's disease, diabetes, high blood pressure and cholesterol, and obesity. Words ending in -ose (dextrose, maltose, glucose) often indicate added sugar.
TBHQ	Tertiary butylhydroquinone (TBHQ) is a synthetic preservative linked to an increased risk of convulsions, liver enlargement, neurotoxic effects, and tumors.
Titanium dioxide	There is some evidence that eating foods containing nanoparticles of titanium dioxide can harm the digestive tract and may induce toxic effects in the brain.
Transglutaminase	This plant enzyme, often called "meat glue," binds ingredients together. People with compromised immune systems should avoid foods containing transglutaminase because it can worsen some illnesses like Crohn's and celiac disease.

THE CALORIES IN, CALORIES OUT MYTH

Most weight-loss diets are based on the number of calories you take in versus the number of calories you burn throughout the day. Under this premise, you could eat anything you want—from chips to cheesecake—and lose weight as long as you burn more calories than you consume. That may sound good in theory but, as anyone who has tried to follow this in real life knows, it's not a sustainable way of eating. You see, when your diet revolves around ultra-processed, nutrient-deficient foods, your hunger hormones drive you to keep eating in search of the nutrients your body needs. But when your diet consists of nutrient-dense whole foods, your body gets all of the vitamins and minerals it needs, so you naturally eat less. This was shown in a small, randomized, controlled trial that compared two groups of people—one group that ate ultra-processed foods and another that ate a whole-foods diet. The study, which was conducted by the National Institute of Diabetes and Digestive and Kidney Diseases, found that the participants who ate the processed diet consumed 500 calories more per day than the whole-foods group. The lesson here? Forget calories in, calories out. Successful long-term weight loss doesn't entirely depend on how much you eat. It's *what* you eat that truly matters.

· ·

Instead of by farmers, Americans are increasingly being fed by food scientists.

· ·

Sadly, these ingredients aren't found just in ultra-processed plant-based meat substitutes. If you routinely shop the inner aisles of your grocery store, you might even find them hiding in your panty right now.

The Addiction Factor

Now that you've seen what these ingredients can do to your health, it's an easy choice to simply walk away from these "Frankenfoods" in favor of healthier options, right? Not necessarily. Food scientists have spent decades learning how to get you hooked on their profitable industrial fare. Like the tobacco industry, the food industry has found a way to keep you coming back for more.

Studies show that ultra-processed foods are expertly engineered to trigger addiction by creating pleasurable edibles far higher in unhealthy fats, salt, and sugar than anything you'll find in nature. Most products also contain rapidly digesting carbohydrates that send your blood sugar soaring. Although that rush of blood sugar can make you feel energized and happy in the moment, it's not long before these elevated glucose levels come crashing down, leading to cravings and an undeniable urge to eat more.

According to one study published in the American Journal of Clinical Nutrition, ultra-processed foods can be as addictive as opiate drugs. Like opiates, these self-soothing products flood the brain with the feel-good neurotransmitter dopamine, which taps into your brain's pleasure centers. Dopamine also interacts with another neurotransmitter called glutamate, which plays a role in habit learning, craving, and relapse. This can create a food addiction that's just as strong as the addiction experienced by smokers or drug addicts. And breaking it can be just as hard. In fact, thanks to the chemical manipulation by food scientists, that old Lay's potato chip tag line "betcha can't eat just one" has a whole new—and much darker—meaning. Food manipulation deliberately creates strong cravings and diminishes the control over consumption, despite negative health consequences and repeated failed attempts to reduce or eliminate intake. And if you shop like most Americans, these food scientists are coming for you.

Can Supplements Counteract an Ultra-Processed Diet?

If you feel like you're hopelessly hooked on ultra-processed foods, you might be wondering if supplements can lessen their damaging effects. It's a question I get asked all the time, and my answer might surprise you. Since I've launched two successful dietary supplement companies, you might think I'd say yes. But you'd be wrong. The reality is, you can't supplement your way out of an unhealthy diet that revolves around ultra-processed foods.

Don't get me wrong. Supplements can be a wonderful health-promoting addition to a healthy diet. If I didn't believe in them, I wouldn't have devoted over half a century to sharing my knowledge on their many benefits. But they certainly can't make up for a steady supply of unhealthy carbs and added sugars.

You've likely heard this before but it bears repeating: it's always better to get the nutrients you need from minimally processed whole food. Although that may be more difficult today than it was for your grandparents, you can still find food that provides considerably higher nutrient levels than anything made in a lab by carefully sourcing the items you buy. Supplements, then, can fill in any nutritional gaps and address specific health concerns as part of a healthy lifestyle.

CHAPTER 2

Dietary Villains

According to the National Institutes of Health, a diet filled with sugar and other unhealthy foods raises your risk of dying of heart disease, stroke, and type 2 diabetes. What do these foods have in common? They all play starring roles in the Standard American Diet (SAD).

• • • • • • • • • • •

But while the government and most mainstream dietitians point the finger at the obvious suspects like refined sugar, they continue to encourage eating other "healthy" foods that, in reality, wreak havoc with our health. Why in the world would they do this? The answer is twofold. First, conventional wisdom continues to follow misguided science that extols the benefits of highly subsidized foods like whole grains. Yet some studies show that a diet high in whole grains is no better than a diet high in refined grains for reducing inflammation. In fact, all grains spark inflammation whether they're refined or whole. However, these "renegade" studies are often buried as the federal government continues to promote flawed nutritional advice.

Yes, it's true that whole grains do provide some nutrients such as the B vitamins, fiber, and protein. But here's the rub: the human body hasn't evolved to fully digest whole grains, or beans and dairy for that matter. Instead of nourishing the body, a steady diet of these foods can actually cause harm and contribute to disease.

Until agriculture was developed around 10,000 years ago, all humans ate a diet solely of foods obtained through hunting, fishing, and gathering. That meant a daily diet based on large amounts of fruits and vegetables, and some fish or meat when available. Studies of the few remaining traditional populations—particularly the Tsimane', Inuit, and Hadza—who eat the way our ancestors did, show that they don't develop atherosclerosis, diabetes, high blood pressure, or obesity.

Despite advances in food production, our genes haven't had enough time to adapt to farmed foods. Add in a full complement of food additives to make ultra-processed foods palatable and preservatives to keep them from spoiling, it's easy to see how modern food has a very limited capacity to nourish and help us flourish.

The second factor that plays a role in promoting unhealthy food is money. The government provides large subsidies to the corn, dairy, soy, and wheat industries, despite these foods being linked to the growing obesity crisis and an array of chronic diseases. What influences these government handouts and, in turn, the government's dietary recommendations? Lobbyists who represent the food industry and the farmers who produce the ingredients used to create the glut of ultra-processed fare. These farmers, as well as processed-food and beverage companies, employ lobbyists to make sure the federal dietary guidelines reflect their interests. While this might help maintain a healthy bottom line for these companies, it certainly doesn't support your health!

So let's unpack the dietary villains that undermine optimal health and contribute to our current epidemic of chronic disease.

Dairy

Does milk really do a body good? Milk and other dairy products provide calcium, protein, and vitamin D. They're also good sources of vitamin B12, phosphorus, potassium, riboflavin, and vitamin A. Sounds like the perfect food. And it is—if you're a calf. But if you're an adult human, it may not be right for you.

One problem with dairy? A large number of people—65 to 70 percent of the global population—can't metabolize the sugar (lactose) in cow's milk. Certain demographics, especially African American, Asian, Latino, Native American, and some groups of people with Jewish heritage, are especially susceptible to lactose intolerance. This can manifest as abdominal cramping, bloating, diarrhea, nausea, and occasional vomiting.

Even if you aren't lactose intolerant, dairy may not be a good dietary choice. Population studies have found that the countries with the most dairy consumption have the greatest risk of bone fractures. In one of these studies, which involved more than 78,000 nurses, increased milk consumption actually resulted in a higher incidence of hip fractures. Other studies suggest a link between high dairy intake and some types of cancer—especially prostate cancer.

Marion Nestle, PhD, author of *Food Politics: How the Food Industry Influences Nutrition and Health*, notes that "milk is not essential for health." That may even be true for children. One randomized study looked at 240 kids aged 8 to 15 who weren't getting enough calcium in their diets. The researchers found that, after boosting the participants' dairy intake over 18 months, there was no difference in bone density between the kids who had more dairy and the ones who didn't.

If you do choose to include cow's milk and other dairy products in your daily diet, there are other considerations. While it provides calcium and other nutrients, cow's milk is also a source of estrogens and growth hormones. Although some of this estrogen is a natural result of milking recently pregnant cows, some farmers continue to inject their dairy herd with recombinant derived growth hormone (rBGH)—a genetically engineered hormone designed to increase milk production. Approved for use by the FDA, this practice results in milk that contains high levels of insulin-like growth factor 1 (IGF-1), a hormone that causes cells to rapidly divide and reproduce. A number of small studies have found that excess IGF-1 can contribute to breast and prostate cancers. However, because this practice and its potential health effects have been widely publicized by the media, it has fallen out of favor, even among dairy farmers who take pains to label their products as rBGH free.

You may also notice labels proclaiming their milk is rBST free. rBST stands for recombinant bovine somatotropin, which is a growth hormone secreted by the pituitary gland. Since rBST also promotes growth and cell replication, it likely has the same cancer risks as rBGH. What's more, since both rBGH and rBST increase the incidence of an udder infection in cows, more antibiotics are used on conventional dairy farms. This means that the milk you drink may contain traces of antibiotics that can, over time, lead to antibiotic resistance.

Thanks to public outcry, it's increasingly common to see dairy labels claiming to be rBGH/rBST free. Yet this may be more of a marketing ploy than actual fact since there are no federal food rules governing these statements. To be on the safe side, look for certified organic dairy, or opt for dairy from goats or sheep. You can also choose organic "milk" made from almonds, coconut, or other plant-based sources.

Grains

For centuries, bread was known as the "staff of life." But today's bread? Not so much. Whether it's made from refined wheat or other grains, modern bread offers little in the way of nutrition. Worse yet, it could make you sick. One of the main culprits? Gluten—a family of proteins found in wheat, barley, rye, and spelt. The two primary proteins in gluten are glutenin and gliadin. Gliadin is responsible for most of wheat's adverse health effects in those with celiac disease.

As most bakers know, gluten makes bread dough elastic and enhances its ability to rise. Gluten is also responsible for bread's chewy texture. But this magic protein also has a dark side—and not just for those with celiac disease. Studies show that consuming gluten can impact the immune system and trigger inflammation in the gut. Since up to 70 percent of the immune system is in the gut, this isn't surprising. Problems can arise when bread or other gluten-containing grain are eaten frequently. Inflammation can then become chronic and lead to intestinal permeability—a condition known as leaky gut.

Your intestinal barrier is the largest and most important barrier in your body. Located inside the intestinal wall, a healthy gut barrier is selectively permeable, allowing only water and nutrients to pass into your bloodstream. It does this by opening and closing tiny canals known as tight junctions. At the same time, the intestinal barrier is designed to prevent undigested food, harmful bacteria and viruses, and toxins from entering your bloodstream. Trouble starts when this finely tuned system breaks down, losing its selectivity. As a result, small amounts of pathogens and other bad actors escape into the bloodstream. Over time, this can trigger low-level inflammation throughout the body, promote cell damage, and interfere with the way tight junctions are supposed to work. While there are a number of things that can contribute to intestinal permeability, one of the most common is gluten.

Gluten isn't the only problematic compound in wheat. Wheat germ agglutinin (WGA) is a lectin that protects wheat from insects, yeast, and bacteria. When eaten by humans, however, it can interact with the immune system and spark pro-inflammatory immune molecules called cytokines. Because WGA can cross the intestinal barrier, it can further increase permeability and enhance the whole-body consequences of leaky gut, including an increased risk of autoimmune disease and cognitive disorders such as dementia and depression.

Another detrimental type of protein in wheat are amylase/trypsin inhibitors (ATIs). Although these proteins also help protect wheat from environmental threats, they've been shown to affect gut immunity, prompting an immune response and inflammation that can worsen intestinal permeability. Research also suggests that ATIs reduce some strains of beneficial bacteria, contributing to digestive problems.

What about other grains that don't contain gluten? Compared to meat, seafood, vegetables and fruits, *all* grains are a poor source of bioavailable nutrients. Some seemingly safe gluten-free grains such as rice or quinoa also contain relatively high amounts of phytic acid—a compound that is considered to be an "anti-nutrient." What makes phytic acid problematic? It binds to many of the minerals needed for good health, including calcium, iron, magnesium, and zinc, which prevents their proper absorption and could lead to a mineral deficiency.

Legumes

Legumes, which include beans, lentils, and peas, are often cited as a good, low-cost source of protein and fiber. They are also high in folate, potassium, iron, and magnesium. So what's not to like? Similar to grains, legumes contain phytic acid. They also contain carbohydrate-binding lectins. Some studies suggest that lectins are toxic and inflammatory compounds that can damage the intestinal mucosal layer and contribute to leaky gut. Lectins can get past the intestinal barrier and may contribute to the development of some autoimmune conditions like rheumatoid arthritis.

Artificial Sweeteners

Refined sugar has been linked to weight gain and a myriad of health problems. So, what can a shopper looking to avoid sugar do? If you think artificial sweeteners are the answer, think again! Most artificial sweeteners work by triggering a "sweet" sensory reaction in your taste buds. And it doesn't take much. Artificial sweeteners are between 200 and 20,000 times sweeter than sugar, without adding calories to your diet. Sounds perfect, right? Unfortunately, these fake sweeteners are anything but harmless.

Like sugar, artificial sweeteners can have a negative impact on your brain. They can cross the blood–brain barrier and disrupt the way your hippocampus functions. Your hippocampus is a key area of your brain that plays a major role in learning and memory.

Routinely indulging in artificial sweeteners can also upend the way your pancreas functions and lead to the abnormal production of insulin. This can put you at an increased risk of type 2 diabetes. And even though they don't provide any calories, artificial sweeteners create cravings, and they can actually encourage overeating and weight gain.

Perhaps the most insidious side effect of artificial sweeteners is the way they affect your gut. Studies show that the regular use of saccharin, sucralose, and aspartame alters the composition of bacteria in your microbiome. In one study that appeared in the journal Nature, this artificial sweetener-induced dysbiosis can trigger a reduction in insulin sensitivity and greater odds of weight gain. Other research reports that the dysbiosis sparked by artificial sweeteners can also increase the risk of irritable bowel syndrome (IBS) or worsen it in those with the condition. IBS can reduce nutrient absorption, dampen immunity, and increase the risk for other inflammatory conditions.

There are several chemically created artificial sweeteners approved for use in low-calorie, sugar-free, or zero-calorie foods and drinks. These include:

✦ **Acesulfame potassium**, sold under the brand names Sweet One and Sunett, can be found in calorie-free beverages, chewing gum, condiments, desserts, ice cream, tabletop sweeteners, toothpaste, and flavored yogurt.

✦ **Aspartame**, better known as Equal or NutraSweet, is extremely controversial. Some preliminary studies linked this artificial sweetener to an increase in blood sugar and body weight. It may also alter the composition of gut bacteria. Aspartame can be found in chewing gum, diet drinks, sugar-free candy, and low-calorie yogurt and ice cream.

✦ **Saccharin,** also known as Sweet'N Low, is often used in baked goods, jams, jellies, chewing gum, canned fruit, candy, dessert toppings, and salad dressings. Although it has been shown to cause bladder cancer in animal studies, saccharin has been deemed safe by the FDA because this finding has not been shown in human studies.

✦ **Sucralose,** listed on many food labels as Splenda, is chemically similar to sucrose (sugar). However, because scientists have swapped out three hydroxyl atoms for chlorine atoms, sucralose isn't digested by the body and doesn't provide any calories. Despite this, some studies suggest that it increases the risk of dysbiosis and gut reactivity. It may also increase the risk of Crohn's disease in individuals prone to the condition. Sucralose can currently be found in more than 3,000 foods.

Unhealthy Fats

According to the American Heart Association, oils high in polyunsaturated fatty acids (PUFAs)—think canola, corn, cottonseed, safflower, soy, and sunflower oils—are heart-healthy fats you should be cooking with. The truth is, these oils are highly unstable and susceptible to oxidation, which can create free radicals that can actually damage your health. Several animal studies have found that these oxidized oils can damage brain cells, trigger inflammation, increase the risk of diabetes, and yes, boost your odds of developing cardiovascular disease.

Such oils are also high in omega-6 fatty acids. Now don't get me wrong, omega-6 fats aren't necessarily harmful—unless you consume too many of them compared to omega-3 fatty acids. Here's why: Omega-6s are pro-inflammatory. Omega-3s, on the other hand, are anti-inflammatory. In a perfect world, your intake of these two types of fat would be about 4:1, omega-6s to omega-3s. The problem is, most people eating the Standard American Diet are consuming about 20 times more omega-6s than omega-3s. And this unhealthy ratio can stoke the fires of chronic inflammation, which has been linked to cardiovascular disease and a number of other chronic illnesses.

Another problem? Oils high in PUFAs are among the most contaminated products on grocery store shelves. Most seed oils are also genetically modified. Making matters worse, many are extracted using the solvent n-hexane—a nervous system toxin derived from petroleum—before being refined, bleached, and deodorized. While this process creates a clear, odorless oil with a long shelf life, it removes valuable nutrients and further fosters the formation of free radicals that can damage your cells.

SATURATED FAT? NOT SO BAD!

Long vilified by cardiologists and dietitians alike, saturated fat was found to have no association to heart disease, according to a large meta-analysis of prospective studies involving close to 350,000 participants.

PRESERVATIVES AND ADDITIVES— WHAT TO WATCH OUT FOR

There's an urban legend that Twinkies last forever without going bad. While that's not exactly true (according to the manufacturer, they stay good for only about 45 days), what gives them the ability to sit on store shelves for weeks and still be edible? Chemical preservatives and additives. Most foods found in the inner aisles of grocery stores typically contain an alphabet soup's worth of these dubious chemicals. For instance, that soft and comforting loaf of white bread can harbor more than 30 different chemicals—from dough conditioners to preservatives—to help create a uniform product that stays "fresh."

Used to extend freshness or enhance the flavor, texture, or appearance of a product, many of these additives have been linked to adverse health effects. Here are the top nine additives to avoid:

1. **Artificial flavoring.** Designed to mimic natural flavors, these chemicals may adversely affect red blood cell production and damage bone marrow cells, according to animal studies suggest.

2. **Artificial colors.** These synthetic dyes, especially Blue 1 and 2, Red 3, and Yellow 6, may be carcinogenic. There is also some evidence that artificial colors contribute to hyperactivity in children, particularly those with ADHD.

3. **BHA and BHT.** These two chemicals prevent changes in the color, smell, and taste of baked goods and packaged foods. Some studies have shown BHA to be carcinogenic.

4. **Carrageenan.** Derived from seaweed, carrageenan is used as a thickener and an emulsifier in some plant-based cheese and milk, cottage cheese, ice cream, and nondairy coffee creamers. It has been found to spark inflammation and contribute to leaky gut. There's also some evidence carrageenan can impair glucose tolerance and insulin signaling.

5. **Monosodium glutamate (MSG).** Often found in canned soups, frozen dinners, and salty snacks, MSG intensifies the flavor of processed food. Research shows that it can temporarily elevate blood pressure and cause headaches and muscle sensitivity.

6. **Sodium benzoate.** Often found in carbonated drinks, condiments, fruit juices, pickles, and salad dressings, this chemical may worsen ADHD. What's more, when combined with vitamin C, it forms the carcinogen benzene.

7. **Sodium nitrite.** This preservative is found in bacon, hot dogs, and other cured meats. Studies show that nitrites increase the risk of cancer because they can form carcinogenic compounds when exposed to heat.

8. **Sulfites.** These chemicals keep cut fruits and vegetables from turning brown and prevent bacterial growth and fermentation in wine. They have been linked to potentially fatal allergic reactions.

9. Yeast extracts. Listed on ingredient labels as autolyzed yeast extract or hydrolyzed yeast extract, these chemicals are added to certain savory foods, such as cheese, soy sauce, and salty snacks, to boost their flavor. Yeast extracts are high in sodium and also contain glutamate, which can trigger symptoms similar to those seen with MSG in some people.

AN INSIDE JOB

What happens when you feed your cells this ultra-processed junk food? Chowing down on a fast-food meal or a bag of chips delivers an excess of calories without providing the nutrients found in whole foods. This lack of nutritional information can lead to a buildup of toxins inside your cells that can, over time, trigger cellular aging and disease. But here's the thing: eating junk food doesn't just cause long-term damage; it can also have an immediate effect on cells. Experiments conducted at the University of Illinois found that even a short-term junk food binge can cause a near-immediate stiffening of cell membranes—especially the cells that line your blood vessels—by oxidizing LDL cholesterol.

To put this in computer-speak, when you eat junk food, it's simply "garbage in, garbage out"—the concept that putting in flawed (garbage) data produces defective output (cellular damage). But simply change that equation by inputting nutrient-dense whole foods rich in information and your output will be optimal cellular function and better health.

CHAPTER 3

Death by Diet—Or How Industrialized Food and the Food Pyramid Can Kill You

For centuries, people ate the foods that were available to them. That meant lots of roots and berries with the occasional rabbit, fish, or, if they were really lucky, bison, deer, or elk. Even after the advent of agriculture, people primarily relied on whole foods. Even as late as the 1950s, most meals were home cooked using real ingredients. Snacking was virtually unheard of and sweets were a rare treat. But then in the 1960s, America experienced an uptick in industrialized food processing. Convenience foods reigned supreme and pantries across the nation became filled with overly processed snack foods.

• • • • • • • • • •

In an effort to counteract America's lasting fascination with these highly processed foods, the United States Department of Agriculture (USDA) released its infamous

food pyramid in the early 1990s. While the government's initial intent may have been noble, the integrity of the food pyramid was quickly undermined by Big Food. And that marked the beginning of the end of commonsense nutrition.

Why the Food Pyramid Misses the Mark

Recommendations for what constitutes a healthy diet have been handed down by the U.S. government for decades. In 1916, the USDA created its first set of nutritional guidelines, which focused on five food groups. These included milk and meat, cereals, fruits and vegetables, fat, and sugars or sugary foods (yes, sugar was really considered a food group!). In the 1950s, sugar was dropped from the recommendations when the original guidelines morphed into the Basic Four Food Groups, featuring milk, meat, fruits and vegetables, and grains. While a step in the right direction, these new and improved guidelines were developed during the very time food companies were churning out dozens of new convenience foods. From Cheez Whiz processed cheese spread to Tang powdered drink mix, these tasty, time-saving foods became pantry staples across America. That meant, because the guidelines never mentioned food quality, a "healthy" lunch might consist of a bologna sandwich on white bread, a handful of greasy potato chips, and an apple—all washed down with a tall glass of ice-cold milk. Sure, it technically included all the food groups, but this type of lunch certainly didn't provide the nutrients needed for good health.

The food pyramid we know today was originally devised in Sweden in 1972 as a way to help people eat a healthy diet in the face of skyrocketing food prices. It wasn't long before the concept was adopted by the USDA and quickly co-opted by the food industry.

The original food pyramid was first introduced to the American public in 1992, and it consisted of six descending blocks. The base, which was the largest block, recommended a whopping 6–11 servings of grains and carbohydrates such as bread, cereal, pasta, and rice each day! Sitting on top of that was a slightly smaller block recommending 2–4 servings of fruit and 3–5 servings of vegetables. The next block was broken into two sections—dairy (2–3 daily servings) and protein such as meat, poultry, fish, eggs, nuts, and beans (2–3 daily servings). Finally, at the very top was a small block featuring fat—a nutrient that, according to the food pyramid—should be minimized at all costs. In fact, over the past 20 years, the USDA's food pyramid has vilified all fat, linking it to faulty science that cited dietary fat as the cause of cardiovascular disease and cancer. This belief has persisted, even though more current studies show that it's the type of fat that matters, not overall consumption.

Follow the Money

But it isn't just misleading science. The USDA's food pyramid (and more recently the MyPlate graphic) is reflective of the food industry's lobbying efforts instead of what's actually good for the health of Americans. Indeed, major food and beverage corporations like PepsiCo, Nestlé, and Tyson Foods keep high-profile lobbyists on the payroll to ensure that their interests are embedded in both scientific food research and the government's dietary recommendations.

Another example of the way bad science and industry interests intersect to influence the USDA's dietary recommendations is the pyramid's emphasis on grains. In the beginning, the food pyramid didn't discriminate between whole grains and refined grains. Today's rendition, however, advises limiting refined grains. As I've mentioned, although whole grains are digested more slowly, *all* grains create inflammation in the body. The advice to opt for whole grains is just another shell game run by Big Food.

Even though the USDA's initial guidelines may have been well intentioned, they've largely been co-opted by corporate agriculture and the food industry. Actual science has had little to do with them. As a result, we're advised to eat a diet that's entirely too high in carbohydrates and far too low in healthy fat. The current recommendations also fail to address the nutritional differences between the types of food in a certain group. For instance, the guidelines don't discriminate between beneficial omega-3 fats and harmful trans fats. It's no wonder that two-thirds of Americans are overweight or obese, one-third has some type of cardiovascular disease, and 23.6 million of us are living with type 2 diabetes.

Until the government gets Big Ag and the processed-food industry out of its back pocket, its recommendations are worthless. Since it's unlikely that recommendations based on unbiased science are coming anytime soon, I say it's time to turn the food pyramid on its head!

Corporate Killings

Huge amounts of money are spent each year lobbying politicians and pressuring the folks at the USDA. The goal? Convincing you to buy and consume products that undermine good health. In 2020 alone, these corporations spent millions on their lobbying efforts:

Archer Daniels Midland	$1,940,000
Coca-Cola	$5,830,000
Dairy Industry	$5,437,038
Food Products Manufacturing Industry	$12,000,000
Meat Processing and Production Industry	$4,190,000
Tyson Foods	$1,291,809
Unilever	$11,460,000

With significant power over legislation, major food and beverage companies have an outsize influence on what gets published in the USDA's dietary guidelines, and subsequently, what appears in America's shopping cart. But the harm doesn't stop there. Industry practices aren't damaging just your health; they also undermine the health of the animals we eat and the planet we live on. But as long as the status quo continues to maximize profits, little will change unless consumers demand a healthier and more compassionate food system. As it stands now, the USDA dietary guidelines, whether presented as a pyramid or a plate, clearly show that money, power, and politics are fueling America's duel epidemics of obesity and chronic disease instead of fostering a healthier food system.

The Industrialization of Food

Let's take a closer look at the practices employed by America's industrialized food system. As a whole, modern food production places a premium on profit instead of nutrition, and it will go to extreme lengths to achieve this goal. Our health and the health of the environment be damned!

Here's how the foods we eat every day are actually produced and how they undermine good health:

Beef, Chicken, and Fish. Oh My! When you cut into a nice, juicy steak, do you ever stop to consider its journey from the ranch to your plate? Maybe you should. You see, most of the beef, lamb, and pork you get at your local supermarket comes from feedlots. These intense industrial facilities pack animals into crowded enclosures, often standing in their own waste. Because profit demands that these animals put on as much weight as possible as fast as possible, they are fed a grain-heavy diet. It takes as many as seven pounds of grain (corn, barley, soybeans, or other grains) to create a single pound of meat. Since feedlot cattle gain about three pounds of body weight per day, that's a lot of grain. And as author and food activist Michael Pollan says, "We are what we eat eats."

It's not any better for America's dinnertime favorite, chicken. While you might envision a barnyard full of happy little hens pecking away in search of bugs and other delicacies, the truth is that the chickens used for meat and eggs are raised on crowded and unsanitary factory farms. Chickens destined for the meat counter, for instance, are confined in large sheds with little or no access to the outdoors. These sheds contain 20,000 chickens or more, all crowded together on the floor. They are excessively fed and get very little exercise. Chickens raised for eggs, on the other hand, are raised in long, windowless sheds that contain rows of stacked cages. As many as 10 hens are packed together in one wire cage roughly the size of a file drawer. To prevent them from harming the other hens in the cage, the birds are "debeaked." These practices are so inhumane that the European Union banned battery cages in 1999.

Farmed fish, on the other hand, are tightly crammed into tanks that are often contaminated with parasites and toxins. As a result, research from Colorado State University notes that farmed-raised fish are typically high in contaminants like dioxins, mercury, and PCBs. If that weren't bad enough, most farmed fish are given antibiotics to prevent disease due to their cramped, unsanitary living conditions.

These conventional practices are not only extremely cruel to the livestock, birds, and fish, but they are also unhealthy for the people who wind up eating them. Grain-fed beef, for example, is high in omega-6 fatty acids, which foster low levels of whole-body (systemic) inflammation when eaten in large amounts like those found in the typical American diet. And if meat, poultry, or fish is on the menu, it's likely you're getting a side of antibiotics and environmental toxins with each bite. Fortunately, there are much healthier protein options.

The Fat Fallacy. Ever wonder why fat has been so vilified by the government and the food industry? After all, fat is an essential macronutrient that provides your body with the energy it needs to function. And yet, science has spent years trying to convince you that all fats are bad. And that's particularly true for saturated fat.

Recently released reports show that the war on fat was actually started by the sugar industry back in the 1960s. That was when the Sugar Research Foundation (now The Sugar Association) paid off three Harvard scientists to publish a research review that featured studies handpicked by the sugar lobby. The goal was to take the spotlight off the adverse health effects of a diet high in sugar and shine it on an otherwise healthy macronutrient—fat. What happened next

THE FAKE-MEAT SCAM

Vegetarian meat substitutes have been around since 1911. Back then, these soy-based "meats" weren't especially palatable. But that all changed with the introduction of Beyond Meat and the Impossible burger. These products look like beef, taste like beef, and even "bleed" like beef. But, as you saw in Chapter 1, these meat alternatives are heavily processed and contain unhealthy oils and genetically modified ingredients. For instance, Impossible "meat" is made from genetically modified soy. And according to a lawsuit filed by the Center for Food Safety, a color additive known as soy leghemoglobin, used to make Impossible products look more like real beef, is derived from genetically engineered yeast and has "no history or knowledge of human dietary exposure." I don't know about you, but I'd rather not be a lab rat in the alt-meat experiment!

Although these products are decidedly better for the environment than beef from feedlots, their nutritional profile certainly isn't as healthy as their proponents profess. Here's a head-to-head comparison between a Beyond Meat patty and a grass-fed all-beef patty.

	4 OZ. BEYOND MEAT BURGER PATTY	4 OZ. 93% GRASS-FED BEEF PATTY
Calories	230	160
Fat	14	8
Sodium	390	70
Net Carbs	5	0

(Source: MyFoodDiary.com)

was nothing short of criminal. One of the three scientists went on to become the head of nutrition at the USDA. Once there, he helped draft the forerunner to the federal government's food pyramid. Another of the scientists went on to chair Harvard's nutrition department. These less-than-ethical scientist's resulting influence changed America's view of what constituted healthy and unhealthy food for decades.

Of course, the food industry's influence didn't stop there. As lobbyists promoted the low-fat craze, they pushed saturated fats off our plates in favor of grains. This wasn't because independent science found that grains were healthier. It was because Big Ag was producing too much wheat. All of this excess needed to go someplace, and that place was us.

But it wasn't just wheat. The corn and soy lobbies also had their fair share of bought-and-paid-for scientists who told us that if we were going to eat fat, it should come from polyunsaturated sources like soy, corn, or canola oil—all of which have likely been genetically modified. It might have sounded good on paper since the human body incorporates polyunsaturated fats during cell creation and repair, but here is why that's a problem: Polyunsaturated fats are highly unstable and can oxidize easily when the food containing them sits on store shelves or when they're processed by the body. This oxidation can then trigger inflammation and cellular mutation that may set the stage for cancer later in life.

But there was one type of fat the food industry wasn't about to vilify. Artificially created trans fats. Formed when liquid oils are saturated with hydrogen to form a solid fat, these hazardous fats are routinely used to make packaged cookies, crackers, chips, nondairy creamer, salad dressings, shortening, baking mixes, breakfast foods, and breads. They are also found in fast foods and premade frozen foods like french fries, fried chicken, and pizza.

What's so bad about these phony fats? When eaten, trans fats adversely affect cell membranes and change the way certain hormone-like molecules, called eicosanoids, function in the body. These changes spark low-level inflammation. But that's not all. Numerous studies have found that trans fats raise total and LDL cholesterol levels, lower beneficial HDL cholesterol, interfere with blood sugar, and decrease immune function.

So why do trans fats even exist in our food supply? Because food manufacturers love them. Not only do they help extend the shelf life of some foods; they also improve a product's taste and texture. But while they might keep your crackers crisp and flavorful, "trans fat is an unnecessary toxic chemical that kills, and there's no reason people around the world should continue to be exposed [to it]," claims Dr. Tom Frieden, President and CEO of Resolve to Save Lives. Many scientists around the world concur.

Trans fats are so egregiously dangerous that, in 2015, the FDA told food manufacturers that these fats must be eliminated from their products by 2018. The problem, however, is that the agency gave food makers a loophole big enough to drive a food-delivery truck through. Despite scientists stating that no amount of trans fats was safe for human consumption, the FDA allowed foods containing less than 0.5 grams per serving to be labeled as containing 0 grams of trans fat. As a result, the average American still consumes close to 5 grams of trans fat a day.

So how can you tell if your favorite foods are really trans-fat free? This bit of sleuthing will help you avoid a good amount of trans fats, but not all. Some highly processed foods can harbor trans fats without listing them on ingredient labels. One study in the *Journal of Food Lipids* found that store-bought canola and soy oils contain as much as 4.2 percent trans fats without listing them on the label. If you see the word "hydrogenated" or "partially hydrogenated" among the ingredients, it means the food contains trans fats.

Sweet Suicide. Although saturated fat has gained an unfair reputation as being bad for you, refined sugar's unhealthy status is well deserved. A diet with even moderate amounts of refined sugar has been linked to an increased risk of cancer, cardiovascular disease, dementia (including Alzheimer's disease), diabetes, elevated blood pressure, high cholesterol, metabolic syndrome, nonalcoholic fatty liver disease, and tooth decay. Not surprisingly, it's also one of the primary drivers of obesity. And the more you eat, the higher your risk.

Over the course of one 15-year study, researchers found that people who got 17 to 21 percent of their calories from added sugar had a 38 percent higher risk of dying of cardiovascular disease compared with those who consumed just 8 percent of their calories from added sugar. No wonder the sugar industry wanted to take the focus off of the sweet stuff!

If that weren't bad enough, sugar can actually make you older, both inside and out! According to Dartmouth dermatology professor F. William Danby, a diet high in refined sugar creates something called advanced glycation end products (AGEs). AGEs are formed when sugar reacts with proteins in your body. This creates a hard, caramel-like compound that interferes with multiple cellular processeses by changing the function of those proteins. For example, when sugar cross-links with the proteins in your skin, it speeds up the breakdown of collagen and elastin. This can lead to wrinkles, sagging, and other signs of premature skin aging. But it's not just the tissues you see on the outside. AGEs also undermine the tissues on the inside by damaging your blood vessels, which can accelerate aging throughout your entire body.

A high sugar intake can also prematurely age your brain by interfering with the ability of neurons to "talk" to one another, record memories, and rewire connections after a neurological injury. Over time, this can increase the risk of dementia and other neurological problems. One study of 2,664 people found that those who drank up to seven servings of sugar-sweetened beverages each week had a 1.91 greater—or nearly twice the—risk of developing Alzheimer's than those drinking unsweetened drinks. That figure rose to 2.55 in those who drank more than seven servings per week. But it turns out that sugar can have a more immediate effect on the brain. Research clearly shows that refined sugar boosts the stress hormone cortisol, depletes nutrients, and dampens immunity.

Eaten rarely and in very small amounts, sugar likely doesn't pose a problem. However, food scientists make sure that sugary ultra-processed foods create cravings that simply can't be denied. According to Danish researchers, eating sugar for just 12 days alters the reward-processing circuitry of the brain in a way that's similar to addictive drugs. Several other studies suggest that the addictive nature of sugar could also be an underlying cause of the mental-health problems an increasing number of Americans are experiencing. In one of these studies, men who ate more than 66 grams of sugar a day were 23 percent more likely to experience anxiety or depression than men who ate 40 grams or less. All this added sugar could fuel depression by causing inflammation in the brain, which is common in those with diagnosed depression. Talk about the sugar blues!

One reason that refined sugar, also known as sucrose, has such an adverse impact on your health is because glucose—which is one of two types of molecules that create sucrose—can elevate your blood sugar. Glucose is a monosaccharide and a building block of all carbohydrates. When you eat glucose, it quickly enters your bloodstream so it can be delivered to your cells. Once inside your cells, it's either used to create energy or it's stored to be used later. Eating moderate to high amounts of sugar creates an overload that can't be properly handled by the body. This excess glucose gets stored in the liver as glycogen or, with the help of insulin, converted into fatty acids that are circulated to other parts of the body and stored as fat in your adipose (fatty) tissue. When there is an overabundance of fatty acids, fat also builds up in the liver, setting the stage for nonalcoholic fatty liver disease. Routinely eating sugary treats, or any refined carbs for that matter, can send your blood sugar on an unhealthy roller coaster of spikes and crashes.

Could there be anything worse? Actually there is, and it's the other molecule in sucrose known as fructose. Since the liver needs to convert fructose into glucose before it can be used by the body, fructose is absorbed more slowly. This means that it won't spike your blood sugar. But that doesn't make it harmless. Just the opposite. Studies show that consuming large amounts of fructose can raise your triglyceride levels. It also boosts your risk of developing metabolic syndrome and, just like with too much glucose, nonalcoholic fatty liver disease.

Of course, because fructose is sweeter than glucose, the food industry decided that adding a concentrated form of fructose to foods and beverages was a great way to save money and keep consumers coming back for more thanks to its addictive nature. And because one of the best sources of fructose is corn, this was also great news for farmers. Unfortunately, it wasn't great news for consumers.

High-fructose corn syrup (HFCS) was first created from corn in 1970. Since then, it has become ubiquitous in ultra-processed foods. According to data from Emory University, 10 percent of the average person's daily calories comes in the form of HFCS. This is problematic since studies show that HFCS increases blood sugar and belly fat while reducing insulin sensitivity. Test-tube and animal studies have also found that HFCS induces cellular inflammation. But that's not all. Other studies show that fructose—and especially HFCS—encourages overeating because it doesn't trigger the chemical messengers that tell the brain the stomach is full. As a result, we eat, and eat, and eat. The natural brakes our hunger hormones use to tell us we've had enough fail in the face of HFCS.

Beyond the immediate physiological impact of eating HFCS, there is evidence that consuming this sweetener on a long-term basis is a major contributor to non-alcoholic fatty liver disease. And, when it comes to your liver, the news just gets worse. Research shows that HFCS is also associated with chronic liver-damaging inflammation and the formation of fibrous tissue. In some cases, these can progress to cirrhosis, a condition that can produce progressive, irreversible liver scarring. This sweet syrup has also been shown to increase the prevalence of arthritis and stiff arteries, even in young adults. In addition, HFCS impairs brain function, increases the odds of developing kidney disease, boosts triglyceride and LDL cholesterol levels, and fosters obesity in people of all ages.

What foods harbor the most HFCS? Sugar-sweetened drinks such as sodas, energy drinks, sports drinks, and flavored coffees. But they can also be found in some unlikely foods we don't consider to be "sweet" such as crackers, lunch meat, marinades, and mayonnaise.

Study after study clearly shows that all forms of sugar—and especially HFCS—undermine good health. In response to these findings, the government launched a half-hearted campaign against the added sugars in processed foods. The American Heart Association also got into the act, publishing a recommendation that women consume no more than six teaspoons of added sugar per day and nine teaspoons for men. Despite these anemic warnings, 1 in 10 Americans continue to get one-fourth of their daily calories from added sugar.

But even if you aren't a sugar junkie, it's increasingly hard to avoid added sugar if you shop at a conventional grocery store or follow the typical American diet. While the top sources for dietary sugar comes from candy, cookies, and soft drinks, foods billed as "healthy" also provide large amounts of added sugar. These include:

- ✦ Canned fruits
- ✦ Cereals
- ✦ Cured meats
- ✦ Flavored yogurts
- ✦ Fruit juices
- ✦ Granola
- ✦ Ketchup
- ✦ Prepared soups
- ✦ Protein bars
- ✦ Salad dressings
- ✦ Spaghetti sauce
- ✦ Whole-grain breads

If you're ready to throw up your hands and simply revert to eating for your taste buds instead of your health, here's a little motivation to ditch the refined sweet stuff. Reducing the amount of sugar you consume—even if you continue to eat the same number of calories—can lower your cholesterol, blood pressure, and other cardiovascular and metabolic markers in as little as 10 days.

According to the National Cancer Institute, the average adult male consumes about 24 teaspoons of added sugar per day. Other scientists estimate that the average American eats a whopping 152 pounds of sugar each year. That's per person!

SUGAR BY ANY OTHER NAME

The only way to ensure the foods you buy aren't packed with HFCS or other added sugars is to read the labels. That's easier said than done. But it's true, you can now see how much added sugar is in a packaged food by checking the nutrition label. The label will list "Total Sugars," which includes the natural sugars found in a food, as well as how much of that total is made up of "Added Sugars." But to discover where the added sugars come from, you'll have to look at the ingredients. And that's a task rife with frustration. Why? Because food manufacturers are nothing if not creative when naming the various types of sugar. Instead of simply listing sugar, food companies can use any one of 61 different names on ingredient labels to denote the sweet stuff. This is specifically designed to confuse consumers and reduce the odds of recognition. Here are the misleading names that denote sugar in the packaged and ultra-processed foods on grocery-store shelves:

1. Agave nectar
2. Barbados sugar
3. Barley malt
4. Barley malt syrup
5. Beet sugar
6. Brown sugar
7. Buttered syrup
8. Cane juice
9. Cane juice crystals
10. Cane sugar
11. Caramel
12. Carob syrup
13. Castor sugar
14. Coconut palm sugar
15. Coconut sugar
16. Confectioners' sugar
17. Corn sweetener
18. Corn syrup
19. Corn syrup solids
20. Date sugar
21. Dehydrated cane juice
22. Demerara sugar
23. Dextrin
24. Dextrose
25. Evaporated cane juice
26. Free-flowing brown sugar
27. Fructose
28. Fruit juice
29. Fruit juice concentrate
30. Glucose
31. Glucose solids
32. Golden sugar
33. Golden syrup
34. Grape sugar
35. HFCS (high-fructose corn syrup)
36. Honey
37. Icing sugar
38. Invert sugar
39. Malt syrup
40. Maltodextrin
41. Maltol
42. Maltose
43. Mannose
44. Maple syrup
45. Molasses
46. Muscovado
47. Palm sugar
48. Panocha
49. Powdered sugar
50. Raw sugar
51. Refiners' syrup (or sirup)
52. Rice syrup
53. Saccharose
54. Sorghum syrup
55. Sucrose
56. Sugar (granulated)
57. Sweet sorghum
58. Syrup
59. Treacle
60. Turbinado sugar
61. Yellow sugar

CHAPTER 4

Was It Something You Ate?

By now, you're probably all too aware that eating a steady diet of ultra-processed foods can lead to a host of health problems. But some people don't need to wait years for problems to occur. For some, food sensitivities can trigger an array of symptoms, such as recurring brain fog, frequent abdominal issues, a persistent stuffy nose, or a mysterious skin rash.

• • • • • • • • • •

Unfortunately, uncovering food sensitivities can be challenging. Seeking help from mainstream medicine can send someone with food sensitivities down one pointless rabbit hole after another. This is because most conventional health-care providers don't understand how foods not typically classified as allergens can trigger such diverse—and often delayed—symptoms. As a result, they may dismiss patients' complaints or try to treat symptoms with prescription drugs. But if the patients are still eating the same problematic foods, their symptoms won't go away—and they may even get worse.

That's what happened to a friend of mine. Out of the blue, she developed tiny blisters and peeling skin on her hands and feet. Her primary doctor had no answers. Neither did the specialists she consulted. In fact, one dermatologist told her it was simply a severe case of dry skin and advised wearing rubber gloves when showering! It took 10 years and a food-sensitivity test to discover the true culprit behind her skin issues. It turned out that my friend has a non-celiac gluten sensitivity. As soon as she eliminated all bread, pasta, and other sources of gluten from her diet, her symptoms disappeared.

It's likely that you or someone you know suffers from some type of food sensitivity. That's not surprising since up to 20 percent of adults in the U.S. are sensitive to one or more foods. And of those, women appear more likely than men to be affected by food sensitivities. If you think a food sensitivity is at the root of your symptoms, consider seeking the help of a functional-medicine doctor or an integrative physician. Unlike conventional doctors, these health-care providers don't simply treat symptoms. Instead, they suss out the root cause of a patient's health problems. That can be helpful since food sensitivities are often a common underlying cause of a host of seemingly unrelated health issues.

You can also take matters into your own hands. Elimination diets or food-sensitivity tests can help uncover the source of your symptoms. But first, let's take a closer look at how food sensitivities differ from a food allergy or intolerance.

What's in a Name?

Although the terms are often used interchangeably, food allergies, food sensitivities, and food intolerances are not the same thing.

Food Allergies

A food allergy sparks an immune system reaction to a protein found in one of just eight foods: cow's milk, eggs, fish, peanuts, tree nuts, shellfish, soy, and wheat. If you eat a food you are allergic to, your immune system sees the allergen as a threat and mounts an immediate response via an inflammatory pathway called IgE (immunoglobulin E). Eating even tiny amounts of a food allergen can trigger acute skin or respiratory symptoms. Some of these reactions can be relatively mild like itchiness or tingling in the mouth. Some reactions, however, can be severe, including a sudden swelling of the mouth or throat, or breathing problems. At its worst, a food allergy can provoke anaphylactic shock, a condition that can be fatal.

Discovering a true food allergy requires testing by a physician and can involve either a skin scratch test, an oral food challenge, or a blood test. If a food allergy is identified, your doctor may prescribe an auto-injector like an EpiPen and instruct you to carry it at all times in case of accidental exposure to the allergen.

Food Sensitivities

Food sensitivities also involve the immune system, but they initiate a completely different inflammatory pathway called IgG (immunoglobulin G). And the root of this inflammatory response may lie in your gut. Recent research has linked the development of food sensitivities to microbial dysbiosis, which sparks the immune response and subsequent inflammation. What's more, unlike a true food allergy, food sensitivities can activate one important type of immune cell, called leukocytes, and cause a delayed response. This means symptoms can occur hours or even days after the offending food is eaten. There's also some evidence that food sensitivities can interfere with the body's ability to absorb nutrients from food.

Another thing that sets food sensitivities apart is that a person can be sensitive to *any* food, even foods shown to be healthy. In fact, it's not unusual to be sensitive to more than one food. My friend, for instance, wasn't just sensitive to gluten. According to her food-sensitivity test, she was severely sensitive to 7 foods and moderately or mildly sensitive to another 78 foods, ranging from bananas to lentils!

Food Intolerances

People with a food intolerance often complain that certain foods like onions, cruciferous vegetables, or dairy don't "agree" with them. Indeed, eating an offending food can cause digestive upset shortly after eating it. While a food intolerance doesn't involve the immune system, it does stem from a lack of the digestive enzymes needed to break down certain foods. Because of this, food intolerances are dose dependent. The more you eat, the worse your symptoms.

Dairy is one of the most commonly cited foods that people are intolerant to. I know because I'm one of those people. Approximately 65 percent of the world's population has a reduced ability to digest lactose—the type of sugar found in milk and milk products. Among adults, lactose intolerance is most common in people of East Asian descent, which includes people of Chinese, Japanese, and Korean heritage. Other populations affected by a lactose intolerance include people of West African, Arab, Jewish, Greek, and Italian descent. But if you don't fall into one of these demographics, don't think you're home free. As you age, your ability to digest dairy decreases. That's because your body makes less of the enzyme needed to process lactose. Research reports that only about 35 percent of people can digest lactose after the age of eight.

If you suffer from food intolerances, consider avoiding the dietary offenders or try taking a comprehensive digestive-enzyme supplement. Check the Supplement Facts label to ensure your enzyme blend contains a full complement of the primary enzymes needed to break down most foods. These include amylase, which breaks down carbs and starches; lactase,

which helps digest dairy; lipase, which processes fats; and protease, which deals with protein. You can also obtain digestive enzymes from some foods, including:

AMYLASE	LACTASE	LIPASE	PROTEASE
Bananas	Kefir	Avocado	Ginger
Honey	Miso	Kimchi	Kimchi
Kimchi	Sauerkraut	Miso	Kiwi Fruit
Mango		Sauerkraut	Miso
Miso			Papaya
Sauerkraut			Pineapple
			Sauerkraut

Are You the Sensitive Type?

Now that you know the difference between a food allergy, food intolerance, and food sensitivity, it should be easy to figure out which you may have based on your symptoms, right? Not necessarily. Because the following symptoms can also signal a food intolerance or allergy—or even a problem unrelated to the foods you eat—it's hard to make a definitive diagnosis based solely on your symptoms. That said, here are the five most common signs of a food sensitivity:

+ Abdominal discomfort, including gas and bloating

+ Diarrhea

+ Headache/migraine

+ Nasal congestion

+ Skin reactions, including blisters, welts, itching, and redness

Eliminate Possible Offenders

Beyond symptoms, there are two ways to determine food sensitivities. The first is an elimination diet. An elimination diet can help determine food sensitivities by removing specific foods or food groups from your diet for a prescribed amount of time. For most elimination diets, that's typically about a month.

One popular and effective elimination diet is the Whole30 diet, which eliminates alcohol, dairy, beans and legumes, food additives, grains, soy, and sugar for 30 days. These foods are then reintroduced, one by one, over the following six to eight weeks to see if any specific food or food group sparks a reaction. Think of it as a highly individualized scientific study in which you are the only—and the most important—subject. As a bonus, while you travel through your Whole30 journey, you may even be able to break long-term addictions to harmful substances like sugar.

Of course there are plenty of other elimination diets, such as AIP (autoimmune protocol), low FODMAP (fermentable oligosaccharides, disaccharides, monosaccharides and polyols), nightshade-restrictive, and paleo. If you aren't sure which elimination diet is right for you, it's wise to consult with a health-care provider experienced with food sensitivities.

A carefully planned short-term elimination diet is generally safe for most people. However, if you suffer from nutritional deficiencies or have an eating disorder like anorexia or bulimia, it's best to opt for a food-sensitivity test to find the root of your symptoms.

Food-Sensitivity Tests

Don't want to spend weeks doing an elimination-and-reintroduction diet? Food-sensitivity testing might be right for you. These tests have the ability to quickly analyze many foods for an IgG reaction based on just one blood sample. And unlike an elimination diet, food-sensitivity testing can help quickly identify specific foods that may be causing your symptoms. What's more, some food-sensitivity tests can be ordered directly by consumers so you don't need a prescription from your health-care provider.

But for all their benefits, food-sensitivity tests do have some drawbacks. First, they can be expensive—prices can range from $100 to more than $2,000—and they are often not covered by health insurance. That said, some tests may be eligible under Flexible Spending Account (FSA) or Health Savings Account (HSA) plans. If you are paying out of pocket, be aware that the price is often based on the type of technology used and the number of foods tested.

Currently, there are two primary ways to test for food sensitivities: IgG testing and cell-based testing. Many popular home-based tests require you to conduct a finger prick to collect a blood sample that you mail in. Your blood is then used to measure IgG antibodies against a variety of foods. According to researchers at Johns Hopkins University School of Medicine, testing for IgG can provide clinically meaningful results.

Cell-based testing is another option. These include the antigen leukocyte cellular antibody test (ALCAT) and the mediator release test (MRT). Although both types of testing look for changes to your white blood cells in response to certain food antigens, they do so in different ways. The ALCAT test identifies foods that trigger the release of DNA by a specific type of white blood cell. During one study, investigators found that ALCAT correctly identified a genetic mutation in people with insulin resistance, which signaled a sensitivity to sugar. Another study reported that the ALCAT test was spot-on for determining non-celiac gluten sensitivity. On the other hand, MRT measures the levels of immune-cell mediators, such as cytokines, histamine, leukotrienes, and prostaglandins, that are directly associated with inflammation. Research reports that MRT testing has a 94.5 percent sensitivity for identifying cellular reactions to harmful antigens that can signal a food sensitivity.

If you're on the fence between testing or simply doing an elimination diet, I believe that food-sensitivity testing can provide more accurate clues to the underlying cause of your symptoms. This can be particularly beneficial if your symptoms don't occur until several days after a sensitizing food is eaten. Another consideration? Even though some food-sensitivity tests don't require that you work with a health-care practitioner, doing so may help you choose the best test for your individual situation. A knowledgeable health-care provider can also help you put the test's findings into practice.

CHOOSING THE BEST FOOD-SENSITIVITY TEST FOR YOU

There are numerous food-sensitivity tests on the market. Most of them require that you continue to eat potentially sensitizing foods in order to obtain accurate results. Here are four of the most popular and effective tests currently on the market:

Cell Science Systems. This ALCAT test measures cellular reactions to more than 450 substances, including foods, food additives and preservatives, herbs, and environmental chemicals. It can be either ordered by your health-care practitioner or purchased directly by consumers. ALCAT requires a blood draw conducted by a lab. The sample is then shipped to the Cell Science Systems lab within 72 hours. Results are presented in an easy-to-read color-coded format telling you which foods elicit a severe, moderate, or mild reaction. Users also have the option of taking part in a 30-minute phone or video call to answer any questions about how to implement the test results. Plus, Cell Science Systems offers meal-planning help that takes your results into account via its sister company, PreviMedica.

Everlywell. This popular at-home IgG test requires a simple finger prick to provide blood for testing. Everlywell offers two food-sensitivity tests. Its basic test checks your immune response to just 96 foods. However, the company also offers a comprehensive test that expands the original 96 foods to include a total of 204 foods. Results are available via a secure online portal. Foods are rated on a scale of 0 (normal response) to 3 (highly reactive). Although Everlywell doesn't offer a one-on-one phone call with a nutrition consultant, it does offer a complimentary webinar providing actionable steps to help guide you in treating your specific food sensitivities.

LEAP. This MRT test provided by Oxford Biomedical Technologies is typically ordered by a health-care provider and requires a blood draw by a lab. The test screens cellular reactions to 140 foods and 30 food chemicals. According to the company, MRT testing not only identifies which foods you are reactive to; it also pinpoints "safe foods" that provoke the lowest reaction. In addition, the results come with a wallet-size card with your sensitivities on them so you have a quick reference while grocery shopping.

YorkTest. This test analyzes IgG reactions to more than 200 foods. Like Everlywell, it requires an at-home finger-prick blood sample. Unlike other IgG tests on the market, however, YorkTest offers tests for couples and families, as well as a specific test for children two years old and older. All tests include a dietary guidebook based on your results and a 30-minute consultation with a nutritional therapist. What's more, the tests qualify under FSA and HSA plans.

Note: Some food-sensitvity tests use strands of hair or a cheek swab. However, these tests do not look at IgG antibodies or cellular reactions to identify food sensitivities and may not be accurate.

CHAPTER 5

A Better Way to Eat

At this point, you're probably wondering what you can eat. After all, between the dietary villains that undermine good health, the industry manipulation of otherwise healthy foods, and the foods that often cause sensitivities, what's left? Plenty! But finding these foods and understanding how they can help optimize your health require getting out of the inner aisles of your local supermarket or big-box membership store and searching out unprocessed or minimally processed real foods.

• • • • • • • • • •

Once you do make the switch from ultra-processed, nutrient-depleted foods to the real deal, your body will respond fairly quickly. In fact, trading out industrialized foods for a diet that revolves around unprocessed or minimally processed real foods can improve your overall health in as little as three months!

Why such a radical change in such a short time? Because, just like a high-performance vehicle, your body needs the right fuel to run optimally. If you've been subsisting on nutritionally bankrupt, ultra-processed "foods," your body is likely starving for the critical nutrients it needs to function properly. Once you do give your body what it requires, you will find that your physical health—as well as your mental and emotional well-being—will blossom very quickly. And it all starts with your cells.

You see, the foods you choose to eat can either provide your cells with the nutrients they need to thrive or contribute to cellular malfunction. This is because food is information. Or to be more specific, the nutrients in the foods you eat give the information and support that your cells need to carry out the vital tasks that keep your body operating as it should. Eating foods rich in the nutrients your cells require to function properly will foster optimal health. These foods provide the correct information to your cells so that they do exactly what they are supposed to do when they are supposed to do it.

You might think that giving your cells the nutritional support they need is difficult or costly, but that's not the case. I've been eating a whole-foods diet for decades, and with each passing year, I've become healthier and more energetic. It's as if I'm aging into better health with each birthday. And you can too!

Build a Better Food Pyramid

Over the years, I've devised my own pyramid filled with foods that put good health ahead of special interests. For the first time, I'm sharing it with you.

Let's unpack each food category, from bottom to top, to tease out its benefits and discover how real food can help you achieve your health goals just like I've achieved mine.

Non-Starchy Vegetables

Non-starchy vegetables are typically low in calories and packed with vitamins, minerals, disease-fighting antioxidants, and fiber—all nutrients essential for good health. But if you eat conventionally grown veggies, you also likely get a side of agricultural chemicals like glyphosate or genetically modified organisms. That's why I'm such a strong advocate of choosing organic when you find yourself in the produce aisle or at your local farmers' market.

Certified-organic vegetables are grown without the use of pesticides, herbicides, or

TERRY'S IDEAL FOOD PYRAMID FOR OPTIMAL HEALTH

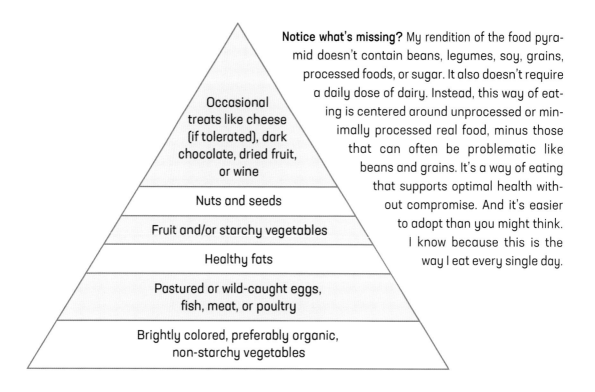

Occasional treats like cheese (if tolerated), dark chocolate, dried fruit, or wine

Nuts and seeds

Fruit and/or starchy vegetables

Healthy fats

Pastured or wild-caught eggs, fish, meat, or poultry

Brightly colored, preferably organic, non-starchy vegetables

Notice what's missing? My rendition of the food pyramid doesn't contain beans, legumes, soy, grains, processed foods, or sugar. It also doesn't require a daily dose of dairy. Instead, this way of eating is centered around unprocessed or minimally processed real food, minus those that can often be problematic like beans and grains. It's a way of eating that supports optimal health without compromise. And it's easier to adopt than you might think. I know because this is the way I eat every single day.

other synthetic agricultural chemicals. As a result, they have significantly lower levels of the hazardous chemical residue found in conventionally grown veggies. Studies show that organic vegetables also contain lower levels of heavy metals like cadmium, which have been found to contribute to a number of health conditions, such as diabetes, heart disease, kidney disease, and osteoporosis.

Choosing organic vegetables won't just lower the amount of toxins you expose your body to; organic vegetables also provide a wealth of nutrients—far more than you get from conventional produce. Studies show that organic vegetables (and fruits, too) contain considerably higher antioxidant levels. One review of 41 studies found that, on average, organic produce offers 27 percent more vitamin C, 21 percent more iron, 29 percent more magnesium, and 13 percent more phosphorus than its conventional counterpart.

Other studies report that organically grown vegetables also boast higher levels of important antioxidants, such as anthocyanins, carotenoids, and flavonoids. According to research in the journal *Alternative Medicine Review*, these compounds are powerful nutritional tools for suppressing the DNA-damaging properties of many environmental toxins. Some organic non-starchy vegetables, such as collard greens, eggplant, green onions, kale, mustard greens, and okra, are particularly high in a certain type of flavonoid known as polyphenols. Polyphenols are especially protective against cancer and heart disease. They've also been shown to possess

anti-inflammatory properties that help guard against diabetes, neurodegenerative diseases like Alzheimer's, and obesity.

New studies are finding that organic foods provide even more benefits. In one recent analysis of 35 studies, researchers found that people who routinely ate organic fare had less risk of developing allergies, birth defects, ear infections, high blood pressure, high cholesterol, infertility, metabolic imbalances, and non-Hodgkin lymphoma.

Switching to organic could also be better for your gut. Emerging evidence suggests that the flavonoids in organic produce may offer protection against exposure to antibiotic-resistant bacteria. These flavonoids—especially those helpful polyphenols—act like prebiotics that provide food for the beneficial bacteria in your gut. Since science keeps finding new ways in which the state of your microbiome impacts your overall health and well-being, keeping your gut in top form matters. And eating organic veggies is an easy way to support a healthy gut microbiome.

With evidence mounting on its widespread benefits, organic is clearly the way to go. "But, Terry," you say, "organic is expensive!" I won't deny that. Organically grown fruits and vegetables can be 10 to 20 percent more expensive than their conventional counterparts. Fortunately, there is an easy way to include at least some organic produce in your diet without busting the budget. Each year, the Environmental Working Group puts out the "Dirty Dozen," a list of the fruits and vegetables that are highest in pesticide residue. The latest version fingers celery, collard greens, kale, mustard greens, peppers (both bell and hot), spinach, and tomatoes. Choosing the organic version of these veggies is a great way to start improving your diet without spending a fortune at your local green grocer.

Protein

I am an unapologetic carnivore. Not for political reasons, but because animal protein—think beef, fish, lamb, organ meats, pork, and poultry—provides nutrients that you simply can't get from other sources.

First and foremost, all of these foods provide the body with much-needed protein. In fact, meat, fish, and poultry are among the few foods that provide a *complete* source of protein. That means they deliver a full complement of the chemical building blocks called amino acids. Your body uses these amino acids to build and repair muscles and bones, and to make hormones and enzymes. They can also be used as an energy source for your cells.

But protein is just one reason animal-derived foods support good health. For instance, beef also provides iron, zinc, selenium, riboflavin, niacin, vitamins

NUTRIENT-RICH NON-STARCHY VEGETABLES

Wondering which vegetables are considered non-starchy? Here's a list of the most popular:

- Artichokes
- Asparagus
- Bamboo shoots
- Bean sprouts
- Beets
- Bok choy
- Brussels sprouts
- Broccoli
- Cabbage
- Carrots
- Cauliflower
- Celery
- Cucumber
- Daikon radish

- Eggplant
- Greens (collard, kale, mustard, turnip)
- Green beans
- Hearts of palm
- Jicama
- Kohlrabi
- Leeks
- Mushrooms
- Okra
- Onions
- Peppers
- Radishes
- Rutabaga

- Salad greens (arugula, chicory, endive, escarole, lettuce, radicchio, romaine, watercress)
- Spinach
- Sprouts
- Squash (cushaw, summer, crookneck, spaghetti, zucchini)
- Sugar snap peas
- Swiss chard
- Tomato
- Turnips
- Water chestnuts

B6 and B12, phosphorus, pantothenate, magnesium, and potassium. And many types of fish are rich in calcium, iodine, iron, magnesium, phosphorus, potassium, riboflavin, vitamin D, and zinc. Some fish—notably cold-water fatty fish like salmon and trout—are also a terrific source of omega-3 fatty acids.

But just like with the veggies you eat, it's important to choose your protein wisely. Different from conventionally raised meat, poultry, and fish, pastured-raised animals and wild-caught fish live in conditions that resemble their natural habitat as closely as possible. It's not just better for the animals; it's better for you, too.

Take beef, for example. Unlike that conventional (and inflammation-triggering) steak you ate in Chapter 3, grass-fed or grass-finished beef is an excellent source of heart- and brain-healthy omega-3s. In fact, meat from cows that munched on grass provides up to five times more omega-3s than you'd get from eating conventional beef. Grass-fed beef also contains a healthy type of fat called conjugated linoleic acid (CLA), which has been shown to encourage weight loss and lower the risk of cancer, heart disease, and type 2 diabetes.

Compared to grain-fed beef, grass-fed meat is higher in vitamins B6 and B12, iron, selenium, and zinc. It's also considerably higher in antioxidants, such as catalase, glutathione, superoxide dismutase (SOD), and vitamins A and E. What's more, it's lower in cholesterol-boosting fatty acids like myristic and palmitic fatty acids. Another plus? Pound for pound, grass-fed beef has less total fat than its conventionally raised cousin and therefore contains fewer calories.

How does pasture-raised chicken stack up to conventional chicken? Meat from chickens raised on pasture tends to be higher in antioxidants, iron, and omega-3s. Eggs from hens given free access to grass daily have higher omega-3 levels plus more antioxidants and vitamin D. And when it comes to eggs, you can actually see the difference. Crack a conventional egg in a bowl. Then break a pastured egg in another bowl. The conventional egg yolk from factory-farmed hens will be an anemic yellow, whereas the pastured yolk will be a deep orange-yellow thanks to the hens' eating their natural diet of grass, seeds, bugs, and worms. And that vibrant color is a good indication your eggs are bursting with nutrients not found in conventional eggs.

Fortunately, grass-fed and grass-finished beef and lamb, humanely raised heritage pork, pastured chicken and eggs, and wild-caught fish are increasingly available due to consumer demand. While they may not have made it to your local supermarket yet, higher-quality protein can be readily found in nationwide stores like Trader Joe's and Whole Foods, as well as some local natural-food stores like Good Harvest Market (Pewaukee, Wisconsin) or LifeSource Natural Foods (Salem, Oregon). You can also have healthier meat, poultry, and fish delivered right to your door thanks to companies, like ButcherBox or Grass Roots Farmers' Cooperative, that consistently source responsibly raised varieties from small family farms.

Once you've found a reliable source for grass-fed, pastured, or wild-caught protein, you might wonder how much of it you should eat to get the optimal health benefits it provides. The average person should consume one gram of protein per pound of body weight. So for someone weighing 150 pounds, he or she should eat 150 grams of protein per day. As an example, that might translate to three eggs for breakfast (18 grams), 6 oz. of chicken for lunch (46 grams), 10 to 12 oz. of steak for dinner (70 grams), and a couple handfuls of almonds and a hard-boiled egg for a snack (18 grams). Getting an adequate amount of protein every single day is crucial for good health. And that's especially true as you age because animal protein helps prevent the breakdown of skeletal muscle mass.

THE PROBLEM WITH PROCESSED MEAT

Ah, bacon! For many people (myself included), cured meats like bacon are a culinary treat. But, like other processed meats, bacon has a dark side. The World Health Organization has classified processed meats, including bacon, ham, hot dogs, and salami, as carcinogenic to humans. Studies show that frequent consumption of these processed meats can increase your risk of developing colon and stomach cancers. But, when it comes to these studies, the devil is in the details, and the risk is dependent on the amount you eat. Occasionally pairing your omelet with some bacon probably won't cause any harm. But if your diet frequently contains processed meats, you might want to reconsider.

What makes processed meats so harmful? Look no further than the nitrates and nitrites they contain. These chemicals are added to processed meats to give them color and prolong their shelf life. But the problem is, they can form dangerous nitrosamines in the body when exposed to the high heat of frying or grilling. For those occasions when you want to indulge, look for all-natural processed meats that are nitrate- and nitrite-free. And if you're in the market for bacon, opt for sugar-free varieties, which you can often find in natural markets.

THE HEALTHIEST WAYS TO COOK ANIMAL PROTEIN

It's not enough to responsibly source your meat. How you cook that meat matters, too. For instance, grilling at high temperatures over a direct flame can create harmful carcinogenic compounds known as polycyclic aromatic hydrocarbons (PAHs). While I personally try to avoid grilled meats, if you do enjoy the occasional backyard barbecue, studies suggest that marinating your beef, chicken, or pork in a blend of antioxidant-rich herbs such as garlic, oregano, rosemary, or thyme before grilling can reduce harmful PAHs.

What about deep-frying? While it might enhance flavor, deep-fried foods deliver high levels of toxic byproducts like advanced glycolic end products (AGEs) and heterocyclic amines (HCAs). AGEs have been shown to accelerate aging and increase the risk of many degenerative diseases, such as Alzheimer's disease, atherosclerosis, chronic kidney disease, and diabetes. HCAs, which can also form during panfrying, have been linked to an increased risk of cancer.

So what are the healthiest ways to cook your meat? Baking, poaching, pressure-cooking, slow cooking, steaming, and sous vide cooking are your best options. But, even if you use one of these healthy methods, don't overcook your protein. Doing so can reduce its nutrient content.

Healthy Fats

Fat is an essential macronutrient that provides your body with the energy it needs to function. It also supports healthy cells, provides the building blocks for your brain, protects organs, keeps cholesterol and blood pressure under control, produces important hormones, and is critical for the absorption of fat-soluble nutrients, such as vitamins A, D, E, and K. But, as you've seen, the government and the food industry have spent years trying to convince you that all fats are bad. And that is particularly true for saturated fat.

Primarily found in animal products, including beef and pork, and high-fat dairy foods, including butter, cream, and cheese, saturated fat is supposed to provide a fast track to a heart attack. But it's not true. A paper published in the *British Journal of Sports Medicine* cited several reviews showing *no* association between the consumption of saturated fat and a greater risk of heart disease. The likely reason is that the true culprit in cardiovascular disease isn't saturated fat but the inflammation that can be triggered by a glut of carbohydrates and harmful omega-6 fatty acids. Other studies have also bucked the status quo. For example, one large Canadian study review found that there was no link between saturated fat and the incidence of cardiovascular disease, coronary heart disease, ischemic stroke, or type 2 diabetes. Other reviews report that people consuming relatively large amounts of saturated fat weren't at a higher risk of either heart disease or sudden death.

Despite erroneous, often industry-funded studies linking dietary fat to an increased risk of cancer, diabetes, gallbladder problems, heart disease, and obesity, more-recent research clearly shows that not all fats are created equal and that choosing the right type of fat can actually reduce your risk for these conditions. Healthy fats—including saturated fat—support healthy cells. That's why I consume plenty of saturated fat in the form of butter, cream, coconut oil, lard, and even bacon drippings!

One superstar type of fat, omega-3 fatty acids, can also foster better health. Because your body can't make omega-3s, it's essential that you get these polyunsaturated fats through your diet. Studies have clearly linked a diet high in omega-3s to better cardiovascular health, improved mental health, less inflammation and liver fat, and even weight loss.

There are three types of omega-3s: eicosapentaenoic acid (EPA), docosahexaenoic acid (DHA), and alpha-linolenic acid (ALA). EPA's main job is to produce chemicals, called eicosanoids, that reduce inflammation. DHA is best known for fostering healthy brain function. These are the two types of omega-3s found in fatty fish, grass-fed beef, and some plants. ALA, on the other hand, is solely found in plants and must be converted into EPA and DHA by the body. The problem is, this conversion

process isn't very efficient. That's why you shouldn't rely on ALA alone to provide the omega-3s your body needs.

Anti-inflammatory omega-3s can be found in many whole foods such as:

✦ Brussels sprouts

✦ Caviar

✦ Chia seeds

✦ Cod liver oil

✦ Eggs

✦ Fatty fish (anchovies, herring, mackerel, salmon, sardines, and tuna)

✦ Flaxseed oil

✦ Grass-fed, grass-finished beef

✦ Hemp seeds

✦ Oysters

✦ Purslane

✦ Spinach

✦ Walnuts

Omega-6 fatty acids are another type of polyunsaturated fat your body needs. But omega-6s, although essential, can also have a dark side depending on the ratio of omega-6s to omega-3s. You see, the eicosanoids created by omega-6 fatty acids can spark inflammation, but those manufactured by omega-3s can extinguish it. While our ancestors typically ate a 1:1 ratio of omega-6s to omega-3s, today's ratio can be as high as 20:1 thanks to the overwhelming number of ultra-processed foods Americans eat. And more omega-6s means more inflammation. Fortunately, changing the ratio can help keep inflammation in check. According to endocrinologist and researcher Artemis P. Simopoulos, a whole-foods diet that lowers the ratio to 4:1 can reduce the overall odds of prematurely dying by as much as 70 percent.

While ultra-processed foods are often extremely high in omega-6s, there are healthy sources. One that instantly comes to mind is avocado oil. Although this oil has a high omega-6 to omega-3 ratio (13:1), nearly 70 percent of avocado oil is actually made up of a healthy monounsaturated omega-9 fatty acid called oleic acid. Oleic acid has been shown to lower cholesterol, reduce inflammation, and beneficially influence the genes involved in cancer formation. This makes avocado oil one of my go-to oils for cooking.

Another healthy source of oleic acid that I often rely on is extra-virgin olive oil (EVOO). In fact, as much as 73 percent of the fat in EVOO is made up of oleic acid. But EVOO has other beneficial attributes as well. It's high in vitamins A, E, and K, as well as minerals calcium, iron, magnesium, and potassium. It's also an excellent source of polyphenols that help prevent LDL cholesterol from oxidizing. Remember, oxidized LDL cholesterol is especially harmful because it can damage the inner lining of your blood vessels (known as the endothelium) and contribute to the development of artery-clogging atherosclerosis.

All this new information might have you looking to swap out unhealthy oils for healthier fats. Here are five of the best:

1. Avocado oil
2. Butter
3. Coconut oil
4. EVOO
5. Ghee

LIKE A (EXTRA) VIRGIN

I'm often asked what the healthiest type of fat is. The answer is easy—olive oil, especially extra-virgin olive oil (EVOO). Of course, there are other healthy fats like avocado oil and coconut oil, but EVOO reigns supreme. It's one of the primary reasons why people living in Mediterranean countries, including France, Greece, Italy, Spain, and Portugal, enjoy such good health. Yes, these people traditionally eat more fresh fruits and vegetables than those living in countries like the U.S. where ultra-processed foods are so prevalent. But experts believe that something else contributes to the health and well-being of those living in Mediterranean countries. And that something is olive oil—a fat that is consumed in abundance throughout the region.

What makes EVOO so healthy? It's extremely high in polyphenols, including hydroxytyrosol and oleuropein, that boast powerful antioxidant, anti-inflammatory, and anticancer properties. These polyphenols are also responsible for that peppery aftertaste left in the back of your throat when you consume good-quality EVOO.

According to Mary Flynn, associate professor at Brown University and the founder of the Olive Oil Health Initiative of the Miriam Hospital at Brown University, a wealth of published research over the past 30 years shows that no other food comes close to EVOO for the prevention and treatment of chronic disease. According to Dr. Flynn:

- EVOO is the main source of fat, and a ubiquitous cooking medium, in the Mediterranean diet. The Mediterranean diet is now well established through multiple systematic reviews and meta-analyses to reduce overall risk of mortality, cardiovascular disease, coronary heart disease, myocardial infarction, cancer, neurodegenerative diseases, and diabetes.

- The well-known PREDIMED study—a high-quality randomized, controlled human trial—compared a Mediterranean diet supplemented daily with at least 4 tablespoons of EVOO. The people consuming the EVOO-rich Mediterranean diet had a 30 percent reduction in cardiovascular disease and stroke. The evidence was so compelling that the trial was stopped after seven years when the advantages of the Mediterranean diet became clear.

- The Mediterranean diet is now recommended by governments, scientists, and health professionals as an example of a nutritional gold standard to support health and wellness, with the PREDIMED trial often cited.

- EVOO is now recognized for its health properties beyond those attributed to its fat profile. For more than two decades, evidence has been mounting as to the role of the powerful bioactive compounds in EVOO. It is now well established that the biophenols in EVOO play a key role in the oil's health attributes, particularly biophenols' antimicrobial, antioxidant, and anti-inflammatory properties.

- Studies show that the biophenols in EVOO provide positive health effects, particularly for overall cardiovascular health. As an individual food, EVOO has also shown specific benefit for blood pressure, blood glucose, plasma lipoproteins, oxidative damage, inflammatory markers, and platelet and cellular function.

- The European Food Safety Authority now allows a health claim in recognition of the biophenol hydroxytyrosol and its derivatives in EVOO, especially for protection against oxidized LDL cholesterol. This permissible claim states that "olive oil polyphenols contribute to the protection of blood lipids from oxidative stress." The claim may be used for olive oil that contains at least 5 mg of hydroxytyrosol and its derivatives (e.g. oleuropein complex and tyrosol) per 20 g of olive oil. But in order to bear this claim, consumers must be informed that this beneficial effect is only obtained with a daily intake of 20 g of olive oil.

On average, people living in Mediterranean countries consume 15 to 20 liters of olive oil per year. That averages out to about four tablespoons per day. Here in the U.S., however, most people eat little, if any, olive oil. In fact, even though it's become more popular in recent years, consumption is less than one liter per person per year.

Another problem? Many people think that refined olive oil is just as good as EVOO. But Dr. Flynn notes that EVOO has unique health benefits—and that the health benefits are due to the phenol content of the oil, not the monounsaturated fat content. "This is clearly demonstrated by studies comparing refined olive oil, which has minimal phenols, to higher phenol content olive oils," says Dr. Flynn. "What has not been tested is how canola oil compares to extra-virgin olive oil. As of 2017, all U.S. health guidelines that I know of recommend olive oil (and do not make the distinction of "extra-virgin") and canola oil interchangeably, despite no studies comparing them."

When shopping for EVOO, be aware that many manufacturers mislabel their bottles as "extra-virgin," but in reality the oil is often diluted with sunflower, soybean, or other nut oils, or they're low-grade oils that have been disguised with chemicals like chlorophyll or beta-carotene to trick consumers. To ensure you're getting the real deal, look at the bottle's label for a "batch date," "bottled date," or "harvested date" that's within 18 months. Also, check the label to find out exactly where the olive oil was produced. In addition, the label should say "extra-virgin." Avoid any oils that say "pure," "light," or "olive pomace oil." That means it has been chemically refined. And always opt for EVOO in dark glass bottles.

Once you open the bottle, smell and taste it. It should smell grassy or fruity and have that peppery taste I mentioned earlier. To protect the oil, make sure to store it in a dark, cool location.

When you do find a reliable source of pure EVOO, it's wise to increase your intake by using it for cooking, stir-frying, and in sauces and salad dressings. But to get a medicinal level of olive oil daily, follow my lead and take two tablespoons directly off the spoon twice daily.

CHOOSE THE RIGHT FAT FOR THE RIGHT JOB

Even healthy fats can become unhealthy when you heat them beyond their smoke point.

Here's a handy, somewhat modified, chart of the smoke points for common fats, courtesy of the Culinary Institute of America.

TYPE OF FAT	SMOKE POINT	NEUTRAL TASTE
Clarified Butter (Ghee)	450°F/230°C	No
Beef Tallow	400°F/205°C	No
Lard	370°F/185°C	No
Avocado Oil (Virgin)	375-400°F/190-205°C	Yes
Chicken Fat (Schmaltz)	375°F/190°C	No
Duck Fat	375°F/190°C	No
Butter	350°F/175°C	No
Coconut Oil	350°F/175°C	No
Extra-Virgin Olive Oil	325-375°F/165-190°C	No

MYTH BUSTERS!

Think eating dietary fat makes you fat? Think again. It turns out that eating healthy fats like avocados or coconut oil won't cause weight gain. To the contrary, they might actually help you shed a few pounds!

Starchy Vegetables

Non-starchy vegetables, high-quality protein, and healthy fats form the foundation of my diet—and they should be the bedrock of your diet, too. However, smaller amounts of starchy vegetables, fruit, nuts, and seeds also play an important role.

Starchy vegetables are a great source of nutrient-rich complex carbohydrates. And like non-starchy vegetables, they are an excellent source of fiber. Starchy vegetables include:

- ✦ Acorn squash
- ✦ Butternut squash
- ✦ Parsnips
- ✦ Peas
- ✦ Potatoes
- ✦ Sweet potatoes
- ✦ Taro
- ✦ Yams

Unfortunately, people often avoid starchy vegetables because they pack more calories and carbohydrates than non-starchy varieties. And it's true. Starchy vegetables are higher on the glycemic index, which means they can raise your blood sugar faster than many other whole foods during digestion. But, when eaten in moderation, they can be a nutritious addition to a healthy diet. For instance, sweet potatoes contain four grams of fiber and are a good source of beta-carotene, calcium, iron, potassium, magnesium, and vitamins B6 and C. Green peas, on the other hand, boast seven grams of fiber, and iron, magnesium, potassium, and vitamin B6. They also provide nearly all the vitamin C you need to meet your daily requirement. But the secret to enjoying all the nutritional (and delicious) benefits starchy vegetables provide is to eat them in moderation. Limit your intake to no more than a quarter-cup serving per day.

WHAT'S WRONG WITH BEANS?

Beans and legumes are typically thought of as health foods. But are they really? Beans are often used as a meat substitute because they are rich in protein. The problem is, they don't serve up a complete protein. And the vitamins and minerals they do provide—folate, iron, magnesium, and potassium—can't be well utilized by the body because beans and legumes also contain phytic acid, a compound that binds to nutrients and prevents their absorption.

Fruit

Fruit is often cited as being an important component of a healthy diet. And it's true that fruit can provide a wealth of vitamins, minerals, and phytochemicals. But most fruit is also quite high in sugar—and that's why I limit the amount of fruit I eat. Consider this: One large apple contains 23 grams of sugar. And a banana boasts up to 18 grams of sugar. On the flip side, a cup of blackberries contains just 7 grams of the sweet stuff. Plus, berries pack considerably more antioxidants than other fruits, with the exception of pomegranates. In fact, studies confirm that the powerful anti-oxidants in berries can effectively reduce cell-damaging oxidative stress.

Depending on the type of berry you choose, you can also benefit from some key nutrients shown to support healthy aging and longevity. For instance:

✦ Blackberries are high in manganese plus vitamins C and K. Studies have found that these tasty berries support healthy cognition due to their antioxidant and anti-inflammatory properties. Research also suggests that adding blackberries to your diet may foster better oral health.

✦ Blueberries, especially wild blueberries, are another rich source of vitamins C and K, as well as manganese. They also contain the highest antioxidant level of any fruit. One type of antioxidant found in blueberries (anthocyanins) is thought to improve brain function by protecting aging neurons.

✦ Red raspberries are rich in the polyphenols ellagitannins and anthocyanins. There's some evidence that red raspberries can help guard against Alzheimer's disease, cardiovascular conditions, diabetes, and obesity.

✦ Strawberries are the best dietary source of fisetin, a flavonoid that has been shown to slow aging and protect the brain. One way it does this is by inhibiting the mTOR pathway, which plays an important role in aging by regulating cell growth and metabolism. Fisetin also reduces oxidative stress and "inflammaging" (chronic age-related inflammation).

As you can see, berries really do provide an incredible amount of bang for your buck. Eating them three times a week, like I do, not only enhances brain health; one study found that it also reduces the odds of experiencing a heart attack by an impressive 34 percent. And it's easy to get these benefits by simply enjoying a half-cup for breakfast or dessert.

Certain types of citrus fruit can also be a good fit for a healthy diet. Lemons and limes are extremely low in sugar and carbohydrates. They are also an excellent source of vitamin C, providing up to 88 percent of the recommended daily intake. If that weren't enough reason to incorporate lemons and limes into your diet, studies show that they are a treasure trove of other nutrients, including carotenoids, flavonoids, and polyphenols. And it's easy to add them to your daily meals. Simply substitute lemon juice for the vinegar in your salad dressing, or squeeze a bit of lemon or lime juice over your chicken, fish, or veggies for a fresh burst of flavor.

While berries, lemons, and limes are my go-to fruits, I do include other fruits in my diet because, although they can be high in sugar, they provide an array of antioxidants, vitamins, and minerals. And because they are high in fiber, they are digested slowly, preventing a rapid spike in blood sugar. Which fruits provide the biggest nutritional value? A study published in the journal *Preventing Chronic Disease* found that, along with berries and lemons, apples, avocados, bananas, grapefruit, oranges, pomegranates, and pineapple came out on top. But a word of caution. Most fruit (with the exception of avocados, lemons, and limes) are high in carbohydrates. If you routinely include them in your diet, be sure to track the number of carbs they provide to ensure they fit into your daily allotment.

Nuts and Seeds

I don't often snack, but when I do, I typically reach for a handful of nuts or seeds. After all, no other food packs as much nutrition into such tiny parcels. For instance, nuts are high in protein and are an exceptional source of the minerals copper, magnesium, manganese, phosphorus, and selenium, as well as vitamin E. However, some nuts are higher in certain nutrients than others. For instance, Brazil nuts provide more than 100 percent of the daily requirement for selenium. And walnuts are a good source of omega-3 fatty acids. Almonds and pecans, on the other hand, are a great source of polyphenols.

Despite being high in calories, nuts are also heart healthy and may even aid in weight loss. Just don't overdo them. One to two ounces—or about a handful—of any of the following nuts make a great addition to a healthy diet. Just make sure you choose raw or dry-roasted nuts to avoid the addition of unhealthy or potentially oxidized oils.

- ✦ Almonds
- ✦ Brazil nuts
- ✦ Hazelnuts
- ✦ Macadamia nuts
- ✦ Pecans
- ✦ Pine nuts
- ✦ Pistachios
- ✦ Walnuts

Seeds are also an excellent source of nutrients. Filled with fiber and protein, seeds provide beneficial fats, vitamins, minerals, and antioxidants, as well. Flaxseeds, for instance, boast a variety of polyphenols. Chia and hemp seeds are also healthy options because they deliver omega-3s and a hefty dose of magnesium.

What about sunflower seeds? These popular seeds are high in fiber and protein while also offering respectable amounts of vitamins B1, B6, and E. Plus, they are a good source of copper, iron, manganese, selenium, and zinc. But, when it comes to sunflower seeds, the only way I'll eat them is in their raw state. This is because commercially produced sunflower seeds typically use canola or other unhealthy oils during the roasting process.

Try adding chia seeds or flaxseeds to recipes. Or simply sprinkle some hemp, sesame, or raw sunflower seeds on your vegetables or salads. It's a tasty way to increase your nutrient intake while adding some crunch to your meals.

Treats

Sugary treats and junk food will never find a place at my table. That might sound harsh, but the momentary high you get from these treats can't make up for the damage they do to your health. And I'll let you in on a little secret, once you cut out these unhealthy treats, your cravings will vanish!

What kind of treats do I indulge in? I must admit, I'm a sucker for organic dark chocolate. But it has to be extremely low in sugar and contain at least 80 percent cacao. This tells me that it's high in beneficial polyphenols, as well as iron, magnesium, and zinc. Studies show that high-quality dark chocolate can lower cholesterol and blood pressure, reduce inflammation, balance blood sugar, and support healthy cognition. But when it comes to chocolate, more is not better. Limit yourself to no more than one ounce per day.

I also enjoy an occasional glass of red wine. Wine contains flavonoids, anthocyanins, and other powerful antioxidants, the best-known being resveratrol. Studies suggest that both red and white wine decrease inflammation, lower blood pressure, reduce the risk of depression, promote a healthy microbiome, and support longevity. Yet most of the domestic wines available in the U.S. contain pesticide residue and added sulfites. To avoid this, I always look for either organic or biodynamic domestic wines or wines from Europe, where organic is typically the rule and not the exception. What's more, I prefer red wine since it provides higher antioxidant levels than those found in white. But like chocolate, a little goes a long way. Moderate drinking—about one glass per day—provides both the pleasures and the health benefits of wine without the downsides like interrupted sleep, headache, or an increased risk of some cancers.

Flavor Your Food Wisely

If you walk down the spice aisle at the grocery store, you'll find plenty of herb and spice blends to tickle your taste buds. Yet, if you look at the ingredients in these flavor-filled packets, you'll see that one of the primary ingredients is often sugar. A considerably healthier way to season your food is with pure, preferably organic, herbs and spices in their unadulterated form. A sprinkling of basil, dill, oregano, or thyme can perk up the flavor profile of most any savory dish. Ditto for spices cinnamon, cumin, or pepper.

One surefire way to enhance the flavor of your food is with salt. But like saturated fat, salt has been painted by food industry scientists as harmful. And just like saturated fat, the goal has been to take the focus off—you guessed it—sugar.

The Truth about Salt

They said that eating too much salt would raise your blood pressure. They said that eating more than the recommended amount would lead to heart failure and heart attack, kidney problems, fluid retention, stroke, and osteoporosis. But "they" were (and are) wrong. Salt is actually a critical nutrient needed to support life. Your body uses salt to balance fluids in the blood and maintain healthy blood pressure. It's also essential for proper nerve and muscle function. Without salt, you would die.

How did the experts get it so wrong? They were looking at faulty research. It all started back in the 1950s, when a researcher named Lewis K. Dahl became fascinated by populations like the Inuits, who consume very little salt, and the Japanese, who eat copious amounts of dietary salt. He noticed that the Inuits had extremely low levels of high blood pressure, whereas the Japanese suffered from high rates of hypertension. From that, Dahl came to the conclusion that salt is linked to high blood pressure. But, because that conclusion was simply based on observation, he decided to test the hypothesis for himself. Dahl conducted a series of experiments using specially bred rats. And that was his first mistake.

Because salt doesn't raise blood pressure in normal rats, he created salt-sensitive mice. Of course, lacing their feed with salt sent their blood pressure to the moon! Not surprisingly, this provided "proof" that high levels of salt trigger hypertension—a concept that was, and is, widely accepted. The theory that salt was a health risk became so prevalent that, to this day, it's unquestioned by the medical community. But here's the thing—unless you're among the 25 percent of the population that is sensitive to salt, you actually need *more* rather than less salt. This has been seen in studies of people across the globe. In fact, coronary heart disease is lowest in Korea, where people consume high amounts of sodium.

Need more convincing? A meta-analysis of more than 6,250 patients found there was no actual link between salt consumption, hypertension, and a higher risk of heart disease. Like many of our dietary recommendations, our beliefs surrounding salt need to be reexamined.

What happens if you severely limit your salt intake? You put yourself at an increased risk of insulin resistance. In fact, eating a low-sodium diet can boost your fasting insulin levels by as much as 50 percent while also increasing your cholesterol and triglycerides. Low levels can also impair kidney function. According to an Israeli study conducted in 2011, short-changing your salt intake can also enhance the effects of stress. What's more, limiting the amount of salt you eat makes sugar more addictive. Notice a theme here?

So how much salt should you consume?

Unless you have a salt sensitivity, randomized, controlled trials suggest eating anywhere from 2,600 mg to 4,900 mg per day—which is a definite increase from the 2,300 mg recommended by health institutions. If you're dehydrated or injured, you may need more.

Since eating a low-carb diet, like the one I eat, causes the body to excrete more sodium in urine, you may also need more salt. This is especially true if you engage in exercise or sports while going low carb. It's a combo that can leave you deficient in much-needed sodium. This is especially true if you're a low-carb newbie. In his book *The Salt Fix*, Dr. James DiNicolantonio recommends increasing your salt intake by 2,000 mg each day for the first week and then drop that to an extra 1,000 mg during the second week to offset the loss created by exercising on a low-carb diet. An easy way to accomplish this is by noshing on three dill pickle spears, five jumbo olives, or 12 ounces of crabmeat. You can also increase your salt intake by drinking an eight-ounce glass of water with a half-teaspoon of salt and a squeeze of lemon or lime juice.

But where you get your sodium is just as important as the amount you consume. Personally, I favor Celtic Sea Salt because it provides the highest amount of magnesium of all types of salt. It also boasts 82 trace minerals. Another form of salt high in minerals, and one that's recommended by Dr. DiNicolantonio, is Redmond Real Salt. It not only provides 60 trace minerals; it also has the highest calcium content of all the sea salts.

One type of salt you should definitely avoid is standard table salt. When table salt is made, all of the minerals are stripped out except for sodium and chloride. Iodized varieties also contain iodine, which was originally added to prevent goiters triggered by an iodine deficiency. It's also important to point out that table salt is highly refined and bleached to make it white. And because salt crystals tend to clump together, table salt also contains anticaking agents with questionable safety profiles.

Master Your Macros

Now that you know what to eat, it's time to tweak your macros. Macros are defined as the major nutrients—fats, protein, and carbohydrates—that make up the human diet. I am a firm believer in a low-carbohydrate keto-ish diet. Why not simply go full keto? A true ketogenic diet restricts carbs to no more than 50 grams per day. While that's ideal, it can be a tough limit for many people to adhere to. My way of eating provides a bit more wiggle room, capping the number of carbs per day to no more than 72 grams.

Here's the breakdown of my macros:

✦ 60% high-quality fat

✦ 30% protein from grass-fed, pastured, or wild-caught animals

✦ 10% carbohydrates from preferably organic fruits and vegetables

What does that look like in real life? Here's a breakdown of my typical meals:

Breakfast: A protein shake that contains three raw eggs, a handful of blueberries, one-half banana, a scoop of collagen powder, and a scoop of egg-white protein powder with just enough water to process.

Lunch: Six ounces of salmon, two poached eggs, and a handful of raspberries.

Dinner: Twelve (yes, 12!) ounces of a rib eye steak, a cup of steamed broccoli, one-half cup of pumpkin, and three to four tablespoons of butter.

This is definitely not what the government or the medical establishment considers a "healthy" diet. But remember, these folks have a vested interest in promoting carbs and trashing the benefits of protein and fats.

Not sure you could eat like this? It's not a diet that you simply switch over to in the blink of an eye. I've been eating this way for many years and have gradually optimized my macros and identified which foods benefit my health the most. If you're new to this, start slowly using the sample meals and recipes in the back of this book. I'll bet you'll be pleasantly surprised at how tasty low-carb living can be. I'll also bet that you'll be dialing in your own macro percentages before you know it.

THE DIET THAT ACTS LIKE A DRUG

If you're wondering how a low-carb, keto-type diet like mine can improve your health, here's a great case study. I met Tom while visiting one of my health-food stores. He'd recently had blood work done that showed extremely unhealthy lipid levels. When he asked for my advice, I told him to ditch ultra-processed foods packed with sugar and refined carbs. A few months later, I received this letter:

Dear Terry,

I just had to tell you that I took your advice about cutting out sugar and carbs, and I blew my cholesterol and triglyceride numbers away!

My last physical showed a triglyceride level at a dangerous 693 (optimum levels are 140–150). My good and bad cholesterol numbers were also not the best. Both my former and current doctors insisted these numbers could not be controlled with diet and both prescribed a statin drug, which I refused. Instead, over the past three and a half months, I've cut out sugar and carbs completely! It wasn't fun but I stuck to it.

When I had another blood test last week, the numbers were astounding. I had cut my bad cholesterol in half, doubled my good cholesterol, and drove my triglycerides down from 693 to 138!

A nursing assistant called to inform me that the doctor said my numbers were "good." I would have expected the doctor to call me personally and ask, "How the hell did you do that!?" Obviously he wasn't interested in learning that I did it with diet and not a statin.

All the best,
Tom

Healthier Habits

Movement Matters

It's been said that exercise is the closest thing we have to the fountain of youth. And it's true. A study of more than 52,000 Danish people conducted by the University of Copenhagen found that there were 20 percent fewer deaths among those who exercised compared to those who lived a sedentary life. Other studies link regular exercise to a more than 40 percent reduction in all-cause mortality. Indeed, next to a healthy diet like the one outlined in the last chapter, routinely engaging in physical activity is one of the healthiest things you can do. In fact, regular exercise is so good for you that, if its benefits could be delivered as a supplement, it would put most doctors and drug companies out of business! And yet, despite the overwhelming evidence confirming the benefits of exercise, the Bureau of Labor Statistics reports that only 19.3 percent of Americans engage in physical activity on a daily basis.

• • • • • • • • • •

In my opinion, that paltry statistic is nothing short of tragic—especially when you consider that exercise isn't just linked to a longer lifespan; it's also been found to delay or even prevent the onset of at least 40 chronic diseases. Moreover, exercise is one of the most powerful tools in the fight against the ravages of poor health as you age. This isn't a new revelation. Exercise has been known to promote good health as far back as Hippocrates, who prescribed moderate daily exercise and famously noted that "exercise is medicine." Indeed, nearly everyone can exercise, including pregnant women, seniors, those with disabilities, and even people with chronic health conditions. That said, if you fall into any of these categories, get the green light from your health-care provider before hitting the gym. And be sure to ask what types of activity might be appropriate for your specific health situation.

When you do start exercising (or start exercising more), you might wonder what you can expect. While it's no secret that physical activity can lead to better long-term health, you might be surprised to learn that you can experience some of its benefits right away. The CDC reports that after engaging in a bout of moderate to vigorous physical activity, you'll immediately experience improved cognition, have fewer feelings of anxiety, and sleep better. Over the first few weeks, regular exercise will help improve your lung capacity and stamina, while also helping you maintain a healthy weight. But it's the clinically proven, long-term benefits exercise provides that really contribute to a long and healthy life. As you'll see from the conditions discussed below, these benefits affect nearly every organ and system in your body. And it's never too late (or too early) to start reaping the many rewards of working out!

THE TOP 40 CONSEQUENCES OF NOT EXERCISING

According to findings out of the University of Missouri, Columbia, not getting physical exercise on a regular basis increases your odds of one or more of the following conditions:

1. Accelerated aging/premature death
2. Anxiety
3. Balance issues
4. Bone fractures/falls
5. Breast cancer
6. Cognitive dysfunction
7. Colon cancer
8. Compromised arterial health
9. Congestive heart failure
10. Constipation
11. Coronary heart disease
12. Deep vein thrombosis
13. Depression
14. Diverticulitis
15. Endometrial cancer
16. Endothelial (the lining of your arteries) dysfunction
17. Erectile dysfunction
18. Gallbladder disease
19. Gestational diabetes
20. High blood pressure
21. High cholesterol
22. Insulin resistance
23. Lack of aerobic fitness
24. Metabolic syndrome
25. Nonalcoholic fatty liver disease
26. Obesity
27. Osteoarthritis
28. Ovarian cancer
29. Pain
30. Peripheral artery disease
31. Preeclampsia (a complication of pregnancy)
32. Polycystic ovary syndrome
33. Prediabetes
34. Rheumatoid arthritis
35. Sarcopenia (age-related muscle loss)
36. Stroke
37. Tendons losing stiffness
38. Thrombophilia (a blood-clotting disorder)
39. Type 2 diabetes
40. Weakened immunity

Bone Health

Brittle bones are often considered an inevitable part of the aging process. But, while symptoms may not appear until your later years, deterioration can actually begin when you are quite young. In fact, women begin to lose more bone mass then their bodies can make by the time they celebrate their 40th birthday. Once bone loss starts, a woman can lose one-half to one percent of her bone mass each year. This bone loss is accelerated after menopause—up to three percent each year—due to the abrupt drop in estrogen and progesterone. Men can also start to lose bone mass at around age 40 (approximately three to five percent per decade) due to a drop in testosterone.

Since a lack of exercise is one of the primary contributors (after hormonal changes) to bone loss, it's important to get moving! While a lifetime of physical activity can help prevent osteoporosis in your later years, you can experience some of the bone-building benefits exercise provides at every age. But not just any type of exercise builds and maintains healthy bones. Weight-bearing exercise forces your body to work against gravity and beneficially impacts the bones in your legs, hips, and lower spine by slowing mineral loss. Weight-bearing exercises include aerobics, climbing stairs, dancing, hiking, jogging, playing tennis, and Zumba. Lifting traditional weights or kettlebells can also work directly on bones to slow mineral loss. What about walking? Some studies show that walking helps slow the rate of bone loss in the legs. Tufts University researchers note that healthy postmenopausal women who walk about a mile each day have higher whole-body bone density. But to get these benefits, it's important to walk briskly for at least a mile most days of the week.

Cancer

Nearly everyone has been touched by cancer in some way. Perhaps you have a family member or friend who has battled a form of cancer. Perhaps that person is you. There was a time, in the not-too-distant past, when cancer was an automatic death sentence. Fortunately, a growing number of cancers are now survivable, especially when detected in the early stages. But, even though modern medicine is better at treating cancer, it can't prevent it. The only thing that can is your lifestyle choices—and that includes exercise. In fact, research has found that regularly engaging in moderate to vigorous exercise can lower the risk of at least seven types of cancer, including bladder, breast, colon, esophageal, kidney, liver, and lung.

While exercise, in and of itself, can't prevent cancer directly, it's a key part of the battle plan to inhibit cancer's formation. Studies report that physical activity enhances the immune system, ramping up the activity of certain immune cells known to target cancer cells and fight tumor growth. Exercise also appears to help people with cancer live longer by boosting specific inflammatory compounds shown to block the growth of cancer cells. But it's important to note that most of these studies have examined the effect aerobic exercise has on preventing cancer. In one study that appeared in the journal *JAMA*, physically fit men in their 50s who engaged in aerobic exercise had a 55 percent lower risk of lung cancer, a 44 percent lower risk of colorectal cancer, and a 32 percent reduced risk of prostate cancer. Studies of women have found that regular aerobic exercise helps prevent breast, colon, and endometrial cancers.

But strength training plays an important role, too. In fact, new research suggests that strength training might even have a slight edge over aerobics. In one of the most fascinating studies so far, a group of Australian researchers at the University of Sydney looked at data from 80,000 adults. They found that engaging in strength training was more effective for prolonging life than aerobic workouts. In fact, strength training just twice a week reduced the odds of dying of cancer by 31 percent and decreased the likelihood of prematurely dying for any reason by 23 percent. The researchers did note, however, that the best outcomes were seen in those who combined strength training and aerobic exercise.

Cellular Aging

If you're looking to stay healthy and vibrant as you age, targeting your cellular health is a great place to start. Research shows that engaging in regular exercise reduces cellular aging in two ways—by protecting telomeres and by renewing mitochondria. First, let's tackle telomeres, which, you may remember from the introduction, are the caps on the end of your chromosomes that

protect your DNA. One study in the journal *Preventive Medicine* reports that adults who consistently engage in vigorous exercise have longer telomeres. And that translates to telomeres that are nine years younger than those found in sedentary folks.

But exercise's impact on telomeres isn't the only way that it keeps your cells young. Another study that appeared in the journal *Nature Communications* found that exercise helps keep muscles healthy by directly supporting the mitochondria in your muscle cells. Mitochondria act like little power generators inside your cells, creating a type of energy known as adenosine triphosphate (ATP). Mitochondria also play an important role in triggering healthy apoptosis (the death of old or damaged cells), and they help cells talk to one another.

By working to maintain healthy telomeres and properly functioning mitochondria, aerobic exercise can improve the health of your cells. And when aerobic exercise is paired with regular strength training, the reduction in cellular aging and increase in cellular health can translate to stronger muscles and a longer, healthier life.

Functional Fitness

What good is a longer life if you can't do all the things you want to do? That's where functional fitness comes in. Functional fitness is simply the ability to do everyday movements like carrying groceries or bending over to pick something up off the floor. Movements such as squatting, reaching, pulling, and lifting are made easier with exercise that supports your functional fitness. Improving your functional fitness also improves your balance, and that can help prevent falls as you grow older. Exercises that target your body's ability to move and function in ways that support everyday activities can also help seniors remain independent. According to one study published in the journal *Rejuvenation Research,* "Functional independence is directly dependent on physical fitness." Other studies suggest that simply taking a brisk walk each day can decrease the odds of disability by 28 percent. This is largely because exercises like walking promote improved gait, stability, and balance—all factors that reduce the risk of falling.

Supporting functional fitness with regular exercise—especially strength workouts—also helps to prevent the muscle wasting that often occurs with age. On average, people lose up to half of their muscle fibers by their 50th birthday. And it just gets worse with each subsequent birthday, making everyday activities difficult to complete. But engaging in resistance training and weight-bearing exercise on a regular basis can delay much of this muscle loss and boost your chances of remaining vital and independent for a lifetime.

Heart Health

Your heart is perhaps the hardest-working organ in your body. Although it only weighs between 8 and 14 ounces, this hollow muscle is responsible for circulating oxygen and nutrient-rich blood throughout your entire body, delivering it to all of your cells, tissues, and organs. But a sedentary

lifestyle and aging can, over time, compromise these actions and lead to some forms of largely preventable cardiovascular disease, including atherosclerosis, heart attack, and stroke.

Fortunately, exercise can reduce many of the risk factors for these forms of heart disease. Numerous studies show that engaging in regular physical activity lowers both total and LDL cholesterol while increasing healthy HDL cholesterol. It also helps reduce inflammation inside blood vessels. It's so effective that a study by the University of Pennsylvania Institute for Medicine and Engineering found that regular exercise acts like a drug on your blood vessels, reducing inflammation in a way similar to high doses of steroids. Other findings in the journal *Circulation* show that exercise can reduce blood pressure by an average of 4.3 mmHg.

To maximize these heart-healthy benefits, strive to exercise as much as possible. In a recent study led by the University of Oxford that involved more than 90,000 people between the ages of 40 and 69, researchers found that the participants who engaged in the most exercise were able to cut their risk of heart disease in half.

Immunity

A strong immune system offers protection against both viral and bacterial infections. It does this by creating a barrier against harmful microorganisms. Your immune system then carries out "search and destroy" missions to find and eliminate any pathogens that breach this barrier and get into your body. A robust immune system also prevents dangerous bacteria and viruses from reproducing, and triggers apoptosis to destroy damaged cells that could set the stage for cancer.

Even though this defense system is highly effective, it's not bulletproof. In fact, a number of things can weaken your immunity. One key factor is a lack of physical activity. This is because exercise helps ramp up immunity by increasing the number of immune cells in the body. A good sweat session also enhances your body's immune response by speeding up the antibodies and white blood cells in your bloodstream so they can detect harmful bacteria and viruses sooner. But that just scratches the surface of how exercise helps keep you well. Studies suggest that regular exercise also:

+ Helps flush bacteria out of the lungs and airways, which may reduce your chance of getting a cold, flu, or other respiratory illness

+ Causes change in antibodies and white blood cells, which are key immune cells in the fight against infection and disease

+ May prevent bacteria from growing by temporarily increasing body temperature

+ Slows the release of stress hormones that can weaken the immune response

According to recent findings in the journal *Clinical and Experimental Medicine,* pro- and anti-inflammatory immune cells called cytokines, as well as other white blood cells known as lymphocytes, are released into the bloodstream during and after exercise. This helps lower the chances of infection. If you do get sick, you'll likely experience milder symptoms and have greater odds of a full recovery than those who don't exercise.

Joint Health

Osteoarthritis is one of the leading reasons people quit exercising as they age. And yet, studies show that exercise is the most effective nondrug treatment for reducing pain and improving movement in those with joint problems. This is because exercise increases lubrication to your cartilage, the flexible tissue that cushions your joints and allows your bones to move smoothly and easily against each other. This, in turn, helps reduce pain and stiffness.

While you might not want to sign up for a marathon or dance-off if you suffer from osteoarthritis, there are plenty of ways to add some exercise to your routine. Cycling, elliptical training, swimming, walking, and water aerobics are all joint-friendly ways to get your heart rate up. And make sure to include some strength training workouts that target your lower body. It's especially smart to utilize weight machines as they limit movement and help ensure proper form while strengthening the muscles that surround your joints. This can enhance mobility.

Mental Health and Cognition

If you've ever noticed that your spirits brighten after a brisk walk, you've experienced the mood-boosting benefits of exercise. Studies show that working out on a regular basis enhances mood, concentration, alertness, sleep, and self-esteem. One way it does this is by modifying the chemicals in your brain that govern mood. These include cortisol, endorphins, and serotonin. Exercise also reduces skeletal muscle tension, which can help you feel more relaxed.

But exercise won't just make you feel better in the moment. It's been clinically shown to improve the symptoms of anxiety and depression—without the use of drugs. In one study of 44 healthy young adults with generalized anxiety disorder, eight weeks of strength training markedly reduced anxiety symptoms and severity. Other investigations have found that exercise also improves depression. During one 12-week clinical trial, simply participating in a 45-minute biweekly water exercise class significantly decreased depression and anxiety in 92 seniors. Other research shows that pairing strength training with moderate-intensity aerobics can cut symptoms by as much as 50 percent in those with major depression.

Exercise can also enhance cognition. People who exercise regularly, even those in their later years, have higher levels of certain proteins in their brains that facilitate the exchange of information between neurons. Exercise also reduces inflammation, increases blood circulation, and prevents the shrinkage of areas in the brain essential for memory and learning.

Metabolic Health

Type 2 diabetes has reached epidemic levels in the U.S. Yet clinical trials show that regular exercise can spark a 46 percent reduction in the onset of this all-too-common disease. Habitual workouts can also slash the odds of developing full-blown type 2 diabetes in those with prediabetes by as much as 58 percent. Even a single workout has been found to increase the uptake of blood sugar (glucose) by muscles among people with the condition.

Since both aerobic and resistance exercise increase the uptake of glucose from the blood, combining both types of activity produces the best results. This was shown in a Canadian study of 251 people with type 2 diabetes. Each participant was assigned to aerobic exercise only, resistance training only, a combination of both, or no exercise. The researchers found that a combination of aerobic and resistance exercise provided the most blood sugar–lowering benefits. Other studies report that engaging in high-intensity interval training (HIIT) is especially effective for boosting insulin sensitivity in people at risk of type 2 diabetes and for those already diagnosed with the condition.

Weight Loss

When it comes to weight loss, the old adage is true. You can't out-exercise a bad diet. Losing weight works only if you combine regular exercise with a healthy, nutrient-rich diet that balances your hunger hormones, reduces stress, optimizes signaling molecules, and resets the bacteria in your gut that play a role in weight gain. Yet many doctors, dietitians, and "experts" continue to adhere to the outdated belief that weight loss simply depends on burning more calories than you take in. Now you might think that's totally logical—at least mathematically—but you'd be wrong. According to Fatima Cody Stanford, an obesity specialist and assistant professor of medicine and pediatrics at Harvard Medical School, the calories in, calories out theory doesn't take into account your individual physiology. The type of food you eat, your body's metabolism, and the state of your microbiome all matter for successful weight loss.

Combining a low-carb, whole-foods diet with exercise can encourage healthy weight loss and even help reduce stubborn belly fat. This was shown in a recent clinical trial out of the University of Copenhagen, which found that exercise enhances the signaling of interleukin-6 (IL-6)—a type of immune cell that can either trigger inflammation or squelch it. According to the study, IL-6 also plays an important role in stimulating the breakdown of abdominal fat in healthy adults. Other studies have found that, although spending hours on the treadmill won't result in quick weight loss, working out can modify your hunger hormones, specifically ghrelin, leptin, and peptide YY. And even if exercise doesn't torch that stubborn fat initially, studies suggest that it will help you maintain a healthy weight once you do lose those excess pounds.

Create a Workout That Works for You

Now that you have your workout "why," it's important to understand your "how." Building an exercise plan that delivers results doesn't just depend on choosing the right activity. It's also important to experiment with different workouts until you find one you enjoy and will stick with. After all, you can have the best workout in the world but if it doesn't bring you the physical *and* emotional benefits you're after, you'll likely quit.

How much exercise do you need? According to the CDC, adults should be getting either 150 minutes of moderate-intensity exercise or 75 minutes of vigorous exercise on most days of the week. Assuming you're working out five days per week, that breaks down to just 30 minutes of moderate exercise each day, or a mere 15 minutes if you're doing vigorous exercise. Personally, I lean toward more vigorous activity, but I've been working out for many years. If you're new to exercising, start out slowly. Over time, you will gain strength, stamina, and self-confidence.

Where should you start? Once you've identified a few ways of exercising that appeal to you, decide if you'd rather try a home-based workout or the gym. If you opt for exercising at home, check out YouTube for a wealth of workouts. If the gym is more your style, I would suggest hiring a trainer for at least a few sessions to teach you how to use the equipment with the proper form.

A Word about Cardio

I'm all for elevating your heart rate and increasing your lung capacity by integrating some cardiovascular moves into your workouts. What doesn't float my boat? Spending hours on the treadmill or elliptical trainer. Yes, you're moving and, in the case of the treadmill, even getting a bit of weight-bearing exercise, but you're not building strength, improving reaction time and balance, or maintaining flexibility. And, unless you're going all out, it's likely you're not even getting the cardiorespiratory benefits you think you are. Fortunately, there are much better ways to incorporate cardio into your workouts, such as biking, swimming, or walking. What's really nice about these activities is that they can be modified to your personal abilities. But if you're wondering about my favorite way to sneak in a bit a cardio, that's easy—high-intensity interval training.

HIIT The Gym

High-intensity interval training—more commonly known as HIIT—is a great replacement for slow and steady cardio sessions. Adding HIIT to your exercise routine effectively improves your overall fitness level with a minimal time commitment. Not only does HIIT have the potential to build strength and boost cardiorespiratory health; it might even help you live longer. During one large study, more than 1,500 seniors were placed into three groups. The first group acted as a control and was instructed to take a daily 30-minute walk. The second group was assigned to a moderate exercise program twice a week for 50 minutes. And the third group took part in a HIIT routine that involved either cycling or jogging at a vigorous pace for four minutes, then resting for four minutes. The HIIT sequence was then repeated four times. While the people in the moderate-intensity group experienced some benefits, those doing the HIIT workouts were fitter than the other groups and had better quality of life. HIIT also appeared to provide better protection against premature death.

But the benefits don't stop there. A recent study that appeared in the journal *Cell Metabolism* found that high-intensity interval training caused cells to make more proteins for their energy-producing mitochondria and their protein-building ribosomes, effectively calling a halt to aging at the cellular level. The trial, which involved two groups—those aged 18 to 30 and those aged 65 to 80—looked at the impact HITT and weighted workouts had on their cells. While the younger volunteers saw an impressive 49 percent increase in mitochondrial capacity, the older volunteers experienced an even more dramatic 69 percent increase. Other studies report that HIIT pumps up both aerobic and anaerobic fitness, lowers insulin resistance, improves glucose tolerance, and enhances skeletal muscle–fat oxidation. No wonder I love my HIIT routines!

Although you can create a HIIT workout that relies exclusively on aerobic exercises like running, walking, or cycling at alternating intensities, I much prefer incorporating my cardio into a dynamic HIIT routine that works my large muscle groups and improves my stamina and balance. Typically, I do a two-minute warm-up before completing either a circuit of several kettlebell exercises or body-weight moves followed by a short 30-second break. I then repeat the process as many times as I can. For example:

Terry's Kettlebell HIIT Routine

+ Kettlebell Two-Handed Swing—20 seconds

+ Kettlebell Goblet Squats—20 seconds

+ Kettlebell Dead Lifts—20 seconds

+ Alternating Bent-Over Kettlebell Row—20 seconds

+ Rest—30 seconds

Terry's Body-Weight HIIT Routine

+ Squats—20 seconds

+ Mountain Climbers—20 seconds

+ Push-Ups—20 seconds

+ Side Lunges—20 seconds

+ Farmer's Walk—20 seconds

+ Rest—30 seconds

HIIT workouts are great, especially if you're short on time. Plus, they are fully customizable for every level of fitness. This means that, even if you've never worked out or haven't exercised in years, you can modify a HIIT routine with exercises that are somewhat challenging but not overwhelming. You can also change up the exercises or intensity as your fitness level improves.

How often should you do HIIT workouts? A study featured in the journal *Cell Metabolism* notes that participating in a HIIT routine two to three times per week improves fitness levels and increases the production of mitochondria. But the study also found that these gains disappear if you participate in HIIT daily. What's more, excessive HIIT workouts may increase your risk of injury.

TRY MY HIIT ROUTINES

If you want to replicate my workouts, it's important to make sure you're doing them properly. This not only makes each move more effective but also significantly reduces the risk of injury. Here are step-by-step instructions on how to do each exercise for both my kettlebell HIIT routine and my body-weight workout. If you opt for the kettlebell routine, it's wise to start out with a lighter weight (especially if you aren't used to exercising) and gradually increase it as you become stronger. Repeat each exercise until the designated time is up, then immediately move on to the next exercise. Aim to complete three or more rounds of either my kettlebell HIIT routine or my body-weight HIIT routine.

Kettlebell Exercises

When choosing kettlebells, make sure the handle is smooth and large enough to grasp with both hands. If you're very new to exercising, you may want to opt for a set that provides one 5-pound, one 10-pound, and possibly one 15-pound kettlebell. As you gain strength, you can add heavier kettlebells.

■ *Kettlebell Two-Handed Swing.* This exercise primarily works your back, the back of your thighs (hamstrings), and your butt (glutes). But it also engages the front of your thighs (quads), your core, and your shoulders. Because these swings are dynamic, you can pick a kettlebell that's likely a bit heavier than your favorite dumbbell. That said, it's also important to control the kettlebell through the entire motion, so you won't want to go too heavy.

1. Place your feet slightly wider than shoulder-width apart and stand in a spine-neutral position.

2. Place your arms in front of your body and use both hands, palms down, to hold the kettlebell.

3. With your knees bent slightly and hips thrust back, adopt a squat-like position, but refrain from going as far down.

4. Using a fluid, explosive motion, drive your hips forward while swinging the kettlebell forward and up to shoulder height. You should feel your hips and glutes engaging in this motion. It is those muscles that should be doing the work, not your arms.

5. The kettlebell should then be lowered back between your legs and the swinging motion repeated.

■ *Kettlebell Goblet Squats.* Goblet squats are one of the best exercises to build lower-body strength. This isn't surprising since, like a traditional squat, it works your quads, hamstrings, glutes, and calves. But, because you are holding a kettlebell at chest height through the entire motion, you're also engaging your upper back and core. This simple addition makes goblet squats a full-body exercise that works all the major muscle groups.

1. Stand with your feet shoulder-width apart, your toes turned slightly outward, and a kettlebell on the floor between your feet.

2. Lift the kettlebell to chest level.

3. Slowly bend your knees and lower your hips down over your heels into a squat position.

4. Pause for a few seconds at the bottom of the squat before slowly rising to a standing position.

■ *Kettlebell Dead Lifts.* I like to swap out the traditional barbell for a kettlebell whenever I do dead lifts because doing so is considerably easier on the back while still providing the same benefits. Kettlebell dead lifts work the muscles of your core, mid and lower back, obliques (the muscles on each side of your abs), and lats (the large V-shaped muscles that connect your arms to your spine). Not only does strengthening these muscles help to protect your spine; it also builds the muscles you use in everyday life whenever you lift anything heavy.

As a bonus, kettlebell dead lifts also help build grip strength.

1. With your feet shoulder-width apart, place the kettlebell between and slightly in front of your feet.

2. Get in a squat position by bending your knees, and then take the kettlebell in both hands. Your spine should remain in the neutral position.

3. Tighten your glutes and activate your core as you raise your body with your arms extended. Push through your heels, allowing the kettlebell to rise naturally as opposed to being lifted by your arms as you move to a standing position.

4. Bend your knees as you lower the kettlebell back to the ground, keeping your arms extended through the full motion.

■ *Alternating Bent-Over Kettlebell Row.* This move will help build a strong upper back and core. To a lesser degree, alternating bent-over kettlebell rows also target your biceps and lats. Just be sure to avoid rotating your torso during the exercise. This will help increase your core strength as you row.

1. Hold a kettlebell in each hand with your knees slightly bent. Hinge at the hip, bending forward so your torso is almost parallel to the floor. Make sure your spine is relaxed.

2. Starting with your right hand, pull the kettlebell up into your chest, squeezing your shoulder blade at the top of the movement.

3. Pause, then return to the starting position.

4. Repeat the move with your left hand.

Body-Weight Exercises

Many people prefer body-weight exercises because most don't require any equipment, although you can make some of the following moves harder by adding a dumbbell or kettlebell. Personally, I find that a body-weight HIIT routine like the one below effectively works the entire body and provides a bit of cardio. It's also a perfect workout to use while traveling as it can be done anywhere.

■ *Standard Squats.* Squats are one of the best exercises to build lower-body strength because they involve compound movements that engage multiple joints and muscle groups. When done correctly, squats are extremely safe and effectively work your glutes, quads, hamstrings, hip flexors, and calves.

1. Stand straight with your feet shoulder-width apart.

2. Bend your knees, slowly lowering your body toward the floor while pushing back into your hips. Do not extend your knees past your toes. Simultaneously extend both arms straight out in front of you.

3. Pause, then slowly rise up, pushing through your heels, to the starting position.

4. Make it harder by holding a dumbbell in each hand as you perform your squats.

■ *Mountain Climbers.* This fast-paced move elevates your heart rate while building core strength and working your arms, shoulders, core, and quads. Although this exercise is easy enough for beginners, mountain climbers are also challenging enough for more experienced exercisers.

1. Get into a plank position, palms on the floor, making sure your hands are about shoulder-width apart and your back is flat.

2. Pull your right knee into your chest as far as you can.

3. As you return your right leg to the starting position, pull your left leg into your chest.

4. Alternate your knees in and out as far and as fast as you can, inhaling and exhaling with each leg change.

■ *Push-Ups.* This old-school calisthenic exercise works your entire upper body and core. By raising and lowering the body using your arms, push-ups target your chest (pectoralis), your shoulders (deltoids), and the back of your upper arms (triceps). And because you're in the plank position, they also hit your abdominal muscles.

1. Kneeling on the floor or a mat, position your hands slightly wider than your shoulders, keeping your elbows slightly bent.

2. Extend your legs out behind you with your feet hip-width apart.

3. Contract your core by pulling your belly button inward toward your spine.

4. Inhale as you slowly bend your elbows and lower yourself toward the floor until your elbows are at a 90-degree angle.

5. Exhale while contracting your chest muscles and pushing back up through your hands, returning to the starting position.

■ *Side Lunges.* Performing side lunges regularly can help improve your balance and stability. This lower body exercise targets the large muscles in your legs, including your hamstrings and quads. It also works your inner thigh muscles (adductors) and your outer glutes. Although you can do this exercise without any weight, you can make it more challenging as you gain strength by holding a dumbbell or kettlebell.

1. Begin in a standing position with your feet hip-width apart. Position your hands in front of your chest.

2. Take a wide step with your left leg to the side of you. Both your toes should be pointed in the same direction and your feet should be flat on the floor.

3. Bend your left knee as you step outward and keep your hips back. It should feel like you are trying to sit just one side of your lower body in a chair.

4. Release the position by pushing off your left foot to return to the starting position.

5. Perform one set of side lunges on your left leg, then switch to your right leg.

■ *Farmer's Walk.* This whole-body exercise is very simple, yet it works your shoulders, biceps, triceps, forearms, upper back, quadriceps, glutes, hamstrings, calves, and core. During a farmer's walk, you carry a weight in each hand while walking a designated distance. Although dumbbells or kettlebells are the standard go-to, you can also use cans, milk jugs filled with water or sand, or even heavy suitcases if you're traveling. Start with a lighter weight and gradually increase the weight as you become stronger.

1. Place the weights on the floor on each side of your body.

2. Bending at the hips and knees, and keeping your back flat, reach down to grasp the weights with both hands. Rise up to a standing position.

3. Stand tall, keeping your shoulders back and your abdominal muscles engaged, and walk forward at an even pace until you reach the designated distance.

Stretch It Out

Remember when you were a kid and you could bend your body into pretty much any shape you wanted? Unfortunately, you often lose this flexibility as you age. Stretching, however, helps keep muscles flexible, strong, and healthy. You need that flexibility to maintain a range of motion in the joints, especially as you get older.

Without it, your muscles become tighter and shorter. So when you call on the muscles for activity, they are weak and unable to extend all the way. That puts you at risk for joint pain, strains, and muscle damage. But building overall flexibility is just one of the perks stretching provides. It also helps relieve stress, promote relaxation, and may even reduce postexercise soreness.

It's important to stretch *after* any type of workout. Stretching before you exercise can actually damage muscle fibers, so wait until your muscles are fully warmed up. Hold stretches for a full 30 seconds. Don't bounce as that can cause injury. You'll feel tension during a stretch, but you should not feel pain. If you do, reduce the tension placed on that particular muscle. If pain persists, stop immediately as this could be a sign of underlying damage.

You don't need to spend a lot of time stretching. A full-body stretch session can take a mere 10 to 15 minutes. But make sure you choose several different stretches to ensure you hit the major muscles in your body—especially those prone to tightness, such as your neck, shoulders, back, hips, and legs. Although YouTube has a variety of effective stretching workouts you can tap into, here are a few of my favorites to get you started:

■ *Quad Stretch.* Hold on to a wall or the back of a chair for balance. Over time, you may be able to do this stretch without support.

1. Bend your right knee and grab the top of your foot.

2. Pull your foot back toward your glutes with your knee pointing to the floor.

3. Hold for 30 seconds.

4. Squeeze your hips forward for a deeper stretch.

5. Lower your leg and repeat with the opposite leg.

■ *Hamstring Stretch.* If you aren't used to stretching, your hamstrings (the muscle in the back of your upper legs) may be quite tight. For more leverage, try using a resistance band.

1. While standing, move your right foot forward and tip from your hips, keeping your back flat.

2. Gradually lower your upper body toward the floor until you feel the stretch in the back of your leg.

3. Hold for 30 seconds, then switch legs and repeat.

■ *Upper Back Stretch.* This stretch can be done while standing or sitting on a chair or bench. Whichever you choose, make sure to tuck your chin and drop your shoulders away from your ears.

1. Interlace your fingers in front of you, with your palms facing away from your body.

2. Round your upper back as you press your hands away from you.

3. Contract your abdominal muscles and hold for 30 seconds.

■ *Standing Shoulder Stretch.* Be sure to keep your shoulders down and away from your ears for this stretch.

1. Lift your right arm and move it straight across your chest.

2. Grasp your right arm slightly above the elbow with your left hand. Gently pull on your right arm until you feel a stretch.

3. Hold for 30 seconds, then switch arms.

■ *Triceps Stretch.* This is an excellent follow-up stretch to a standing shoulder stretch. Be sure to relax your shoulders and reach your fingertips as far down your upper back as you can.

1. Bring your right elbow straight up toward the ceiling while bending your arm.

2. Grab your right elbow with your left hand and gently pull your elbow down toward your head until you feel a stretch in your triceps (the muscle on the backside of your arm).

3. Hold for 30 seconds, then switch arms.

NO TIME TO EXERCISE? TRY THIS!

One of the biggest excuses for not exercising is a lack of time. And I get it—life can get busy. But the secret to fitting fitness into a busy schedule is to choose an exercise that works your whole body and elevates your heart rate in a short amount of time. For me, that means two-handed kettlebell swings. It's my absolute favorite exercise when I've got only 15 to 20 minutes because it's highly effective for building your stamina while also working your shoulders, core, back, glutes, and legs.

To get these benefits, grab a kettlebell and follow the instructions in the "Kettlebell Exercises" section of this chapter. For women, I recommend choosing a kettlebell weight of 15 to 20 pounds. For men, opt for 20 to 36 pounds. Here's what my routine looks like when I'm short on time:

- Using proper form, do 30 to 40 kettlebells swings. This should take one minute or less.

- Spend the next two minutes doing "active rest." This could be jumping rope, jogging on a treadmill, or riding a stationary bike (my personal favorite).

- Repeat this sequence five or six times for a total of 6 minutes of kettlebell swings and 15 to 20 minutes of total exercise.

There you have it. A full-body workout in less time than it takes to watch an episode of your favorite sitcom. You can also swap out the kettlebell swings for a farmer's walk (walking 20 to 50 yards per round) or kettlebell squats (15 to 30 repetitions per round). Instructions for these are also under the "Kettlebell Exercises" section. If you're a visual learner, however, you can easily find videos of each exercise online.

DEALING WITH DOMS

Delayed onset muscle soreness (DOMS) is perhaps the most common type of muscle pain—and that's especially true when you first start on your workout journey. DOMS typically develops 12 to 24 hours after an activity that places unaccustomed stress on muscles—and once it hits, it can last for up to 72 hours. One common misconception is that DOMS is the result of lactic-acid buildup. The truth is, DOMS is actually a side effect of the repair process in response to microscopic damage that occurs as you build muscle.

If you experience DOMS, ice the affected area several times a day. Instead of taking ibuprofen—which may actually delay muscle repair—opt for supplementing with a high-quality bioavailable curcumin like BCM-95. Studies have found that curcumin effectively reduces inflammation and increases muscle regeneration postexercise. Other botanicals that work well with curcumin to relieve muscle pain include boswellia that's standardized to contain at least 10 percent AKBA, white willow bark that's standardized to contain at least 15 percent salicylic acid, and devil's claw that contains at least 20 percent harpagosides.

POSTURAL THERAPY

Remember your parents telling you to "stand up straight" when you were a kid? Now that you're an adult, there's no one around to remind you of the importance of good posture. And so it's not unusual for adults to find themselves either hunched over their desk or slumped in a chair after a hard day. But poor posture doesn't just look unattractive; it may be causing neck, shoulder, and back pain. Studies show that, over time, poor posture can lead to spinal dysfunction, joint degeneration, rounded shoulders, poor circulation, fatigue, jaw pain, headaches, breathing problems, and more. While exercise can foster some improvement, effectively correcting poor posture often requires more intense treatment.

Enter postural therapy, a type of therapy also known as the Egoscue Method that helps to correct postural imbalances. It does this by using your own body weight to improve the alignment of the spine and the balance of the body. At the core of postural therapy is the hypothesis that the body has eight load-bearing joints found in the shoulders, hips, knees, and ankles. When these joints aren't in alignment, the body can't perform at its best. Speaking from first-hand experience, I can tell you that restoring alignment not only relieves pain and improves breathing; it can enhance your overall health.

But postural therapy isn't a do-it-yourself proposition. To truly get the most benefit, work with a physical therapist certified in the Egoscue Method. To find a certified therapist near you, check *egoscue.com/find-therapy*.

CHAPTER 7

Get Your Zzzz's

How did you sleep last night? Were you able to nod off quickly or did you toss and turn all night long with your mind racing? Did you wake up refreshed or did you wake up just as tired as you were when you went to bed? The truth is, many of us aren't getting the high-quality sleep we need for optimal health. In fact, slightly more than 35 percent of adults report getting fewer than seven hours of sleep per night. And as many as 30 percent of young and middle-aged adults say they suffer from chronic insomnia. That statistic rises to 48 percent as we enter our golden years. Unfortunately, this lack of sleep is doing a real number on our health and our ability to function optimally on a daily basis.

• • • • • • • • • •

Why Sleep Matters

Have you ever wondered why sleep is so important? Although there's a lot that scientists don't yet know, studies do show that sleep allows the brain to purge toxic waste products and store new information. While you sleep, your nerve cells also reorganize themselves, and your body uses this downtime to repair cells, release hormones and proteins, and refill your "energy tank" so you can have the motivation to do what needs to be done the next day.

Research suggests that sleep further supports brain function by controlling how memories are stored and by purging unnecessary information that can clutter your mind. High-quality sleep improves concentration, focus, creativity, problem-solving, and decision-making. It also helps regulate your mood. Even one night of poor sleep can reduce your ability to regulate your emotions and leave you more vulnerable to emotional outbursts and hurt feelings. Chronic sleep deprivation has also been found to increase the risk of depression. In one study of 2,672 people that appeared in the journal *Frontiers in Neurology*, scientists found that those suffering from anxiety and depression were more likely to report problems sleeping.

Poor sleep also leads to some surprising consequences. If you've ever wondered why you reach for that pint of Ben & Jerry's or that bag of chips after a lousy night's sleep, blame its impact on your hunger hormones. When you're sleeping well, your body produces less of the appetite-boosting hormone ghrelin and more of the satiety hormone leptin. But when you shortchange the amount of time sleeping or you suffer from poor-quality sleep, the opposite occurs: more ghrelin and less leptin. Not only does this increase hunger the next day; you'll be more likely to crave unhealthy ultra-processed foods.

Pulling an all-nighter or logging a poor night's sleep once in a while won't likely cause any lasting damage, but chronic sleep deprivation—as little as five nights in a row of poor sleep—has been linked to greater odds of obesity, metabolic syndrome, and type 2 diabetes. What's more, new evidence from researchers at the Mayo Clinic demonstrates that sleep deprivation not only contributes to overall weight gain; it can lead to a 9 percent increase in abdominal fat and an 11 percent increase in visceral fat. This is especially dangerous since visceral fat, which is located deep inside the abdomen, surrounds your vital organs, including your intestines, liver, and pancreas, and is strongly correlated with metabolic disease.

If you're routinely getting too-little or poor-quality sleep, studies have shown that you're more prone to developing cardiovascular disease. In one review of 19 studies, people who got fewer than seven hours of sleep per night had a 13 percent greater risk of dying of heart disease than people who got the recommended seven to nine hours. On the other hand, getting enough high-quality sleep promotes proper pancreatic function, a stronger immune system, and less inflammation. Plus, it can support heart health by fostering healthy blood pressure.

The Circadian Connection

The ability to get good sleep depends largely on your internal clock—better known as your circadian rhythm. This biological clock regulates your sleep-wake cycle in response to light and darkness. Historically (as in before electric lights), people would structure their lives in accordance to their circadian rhythm, waking with the sun and going to sleep once night set in. Living in accordance to this system worked well for centuries—until we conquered the darkness with the electric light bulb. Today, we can stay up until any hour, working and socializing round the clock.

But this shift in our sleep-wake cycle has a number of causes beyond our extended exposure to artificial light. Other factors that can upend the circadian rhythm include:

✦ Advancing age

✦ Alcohol use shortly before turning in

✦ Alzheimer's disease and dementia

✦ Bipolar disorder

✦ Dealing with changes in time zones (jet lag)

✦ Exercising close to bedtime

✦ Exposure to bright light and blue light

+ Menopause

+ Oversleeping

+ Pregnancy

+ Pulling an all-nighter

+ Recreational drug use

+ Shift work

Fortunately, simply making a few changes to your habits can help reset your circadian rhythm. However, if you have a health condition that disrupts your sleep, it's wise to see your health-care provider for help.

Sleepless in Seattle– And Everywhere Else

Aside from imbalances in your circadian rhythm, other reasons you aren't getting good sleep can include chronic insomnia, sleep apnea, and snoring. Any one of these can result in shortened or poor-quality sleep, leaving you groggy and dragging the next day. The good news is that help can be had for all of these conditions.

Insomnia. One of the most common—and the most frustrating—sleep disorders is insomnia, which is defined as trouble falling asleep, staying asleep, or both.

THE BAD NEWS ABOUT BLUE LIGHT

If you spend the evening in front of the TV or if you climb into bed and immediately start scrolling your social-media feeds, it's time to stop! You see, all those devices, as well as the fluorescent and LED lights in your environment, emit blue light that can interfere with your sleep. Blue light is the part of the visible light spectrum that can impact your alertness, hormone production, and sleep cycle. It's not only produced by your devices; it's also emitted by the sun. That could be why you likely feel more energized during the day, especially if you spend time outside in the sunshine. But mimicking blue light after dark via artificial light or your high-tech devices can disrupt the circadian rhythm and interfere with sleep. In one study conducted by researchers at Harvard Medical School and Brigham and Women's Hospital, people exposed to blue light during the evening hours released less melatonin. As a result, their sleep cycles were delayed or disrupted. In order to avoid this happening to you, sleep experts advise turning down the lights in the evening and putting all of your devices away at least one hour before turning in. Another option? Try blue-light blocking glasses when the sun goes down. During a small trial involving 20 adult volunteers, those who wore amber blue-light blocking glasses for three hours in the evening experienced a significant improvement in their sleep quality and mood compared to those wearing glasses that didn't block the disruptive rays.

Approximately 30 percent of Americans experience short-term insomnia, which typically lasts from a few days to a few weeks. Chronic insomnia, on the other hand, can last for a month or more and it impacts about 10 percent of all Americans. Underlying causes for this inability to sleep can include chronic stress, shift work, and travel. Alcohol, caffeine, tobacco, and a sedentary lifestyle can make insomnia even worse.

Insomnia that lasts for more than a couple of days can interfere with your ability to function. You might have trouble remembering information or focusing at work or school. Or you might feel drowsy while driving, increasing the risk of an accident. Ongoing sleep deprivation can also increase your risk of anxiety, dementia, depression, diabetes, heart attack, high blood pressure, infertility, weakened immunity, and weight gain. While there are drugs designed to treat insomnia, they come with a laundry list of side effects, ranging from digestive problems to mental impairment to hallucinations. Prescription sleep aids can also be addictive. But insomnia can often be managed with lifestyle changes and supplements like melatonin.

Sleep apnea. Has anyone ever told you that you snore or gasp while you're asleep? If so, you might have sleep apnea—a condition in which you temporarily stop breathing while you're sleeping. There are three types of sleep apnea: Obstructive sleep apnea occurs when the throat muscles relax and block the upper airway; central sleep apnea happens when the brain doesn't send the proper signals to the muscles that control breathing; and complex sleep apnea syndrome, which is a combination of obstructive and central sleep apneas. Risk factors can include:

✦ Being male

✦ Being older

✦ Being overweight

✦ Existing medical conditions such as asthma, high blood pressure, or type 2 diabetes

✦ Family history

✦ Having a narrowed airway

✦ Nasal congestion

✦ Smoking

✦ The use of alcohol, sedatives, or tranquilizers

While people with sleep apnea typically don't stop breathing for more than a few seconds, it can have a negative impact on sleep quality. And that can lead to feeling tired the next day. But, because of how the condition impacts the balance of oxygen in the body, untreated sleep apnea raises the risk for a number of seemingly unrelated health issues, including atrial fibrillation, high blood pressure, liver problems, metabolic syndrome, and type 2 diabetes. If you suspect that you suffer from sleep apnea, it's important to talk with your doctor. He or she might recommend taking part in a sleep study to confirm the diagnosis. Mild cases can often be treated by losing weight or breaking habits like smoking or drinking, if applicable. Moderate cases are often

THE STAGES OF SLEEP

Now that you know what can go wrong, let's take a look at what happens during sleep when things go right. Normally, you sleep in stages throughout the night. These stages fall into two categories: rapid eye movement (REM) sleep, which has just one stage, and non-REM sleep, which cycles through three different stages. Each of these stages is linked to specific activity in your brain, and they repeat several times throughout the night.

REM sleep. Often associated with dreaming, REM sleep first occurs about 90 minutes after you nod off. Your eyes start to move rapidly from side to side behind closed eyelids. Your breathing becomes faster and irregular. And your heart rate and blood pressure increase. Your arm and leg muscles also become temporarily paralyzed—which is the body's way of keeping you from acting out your dreams. But your brain isn't just busy dreaming. Scientists believe the REM cycle may play a role in sorting and storing memories, supporting neuroplasticity (the brain's ability to change and adapt to new experiences and information), learning new skills, regulating mood, and even processing stress. But as you age, you spend less of your sleep time in REM.

Stage 1 Sleep. The first stage of non-REM sleep occurs during the changeover from wakefulness to sleep. When you first fall asleep, your heartbeat, breathing, and eye movements slow, and your muscles relax, with occasional twitches. Your brain waves also begin to slow from their daytime wakefulness patterns.

Stage 2 Sleep. This is a period of light sleep before you enter deeper sleep. Your heartbeat and breathing slow down as your muscles relax even more. Your body temperature drops and your eye movements stop. The activity in your brain decreases but you still experience brief bursts of electrical activity.

Stage 3 Sleep. Also known as deep sleep, this stage of non-REM sleep often occurs during the first half of the night. In this stage, your heart rate, breathing, and brain waves all drop to their lowest level of activity. Deep sleep strengthens the immune system and plays a role in the way your brain learns and stores memories. But, as important as deep sleep seems to be, the amount you get decreases as you age.

treated with a CPAP machine. This device is worn while you sleep and keeps the upper airway passages open by creating air pressure that is somewhat greater than that of the surrounding air. Depending on the severity of your sleep apnea, acupuncture is another drug-free treatment that may improve the condition. During one Chinese study of 30 people with obstructive sleep apnea, those undergoing acupuncture three to five times per week (for a total of 30 sessions) showed a significant improvement in their oxygen intake during sleep.

Snoring. If you've ever slept in the same room as someone who snores, you know how disruptive it can be—especially if you're trying to get a good night's sleep. Snoring is the most common type of sleep disorder, affecting 45 percent of people occasionally and 25 percent routinely. And it doesn't get any better with age. In fact, half of all people over the age of 60 snore. That's a problem because loud or long-term snoring increases the risk of heart attack, stroke, and other health problems. Habitual snoring can also have a negative impact on relationships. According to statistics, it's the third leading cause of divorce!

Snoring is caused by the vibration of tissues in the back of the throat near the airway. Inhaling and exhaling as you sleep can cause these tissues to "flutter" and make a noise like a flag being whipped around by the wind. If you do snore, even occasionally, there are a number of natural lifestyle changes that may help you stop. These include:

+ Avoiding alcohol or sedatives several hours before turning in
+ Losing weight if needed
+ Raising the head of your bed
+ Sleeping on your side
+ Stopping smoking if applicable
+ Using breathing strips to open your nasal passages

Adopt These Healthy Sleep Habits

I travel often for both work and pleasure. And my travels can frequently put me in such far-flung places as India, Venice, or Paris. While I love exploring all the world has to offer, the change in time zones can be a challenge. Fortunately, I've learned some tricks for getting good sleep, whether I'm at home or on the road. Here are some of my favorite "sleep hacks" that might help you get a better night's sleep, too.

+ Avoid caffeine at least six to eight hours before turning in.
+ Create a wind-down routine that might include meditating, journaling, stretching, or a warm bath.
+ Design a calming sleep environment that includes soft non-LED lighting, soothing colors, cozy bedding, and a comfortable mattress.
+ Don't eat within three hours of your normal bedtime.

✦ Exercise daily, but no later than three or four hours before going to bed.

✦ If ambient light is a problem, try wearing a light-blocking sleep mask or consider blackout curtains.

✦ Limit your alcohol intake and don't indulge before bed.

✦ Remove all screens (TV, laptop, mobile phone, etc.) from your bedroom.

✦ Reserve your bedroom for sleep and sex—nothing else.

✦ Set a consistent sleep schedule, going to bed and waking up at the same time each day.

✦ Turn the thermostat down to 68° to foster better sleep.

If, despite trying these strategies, you still can't sleep, don't lie in bed awake. If you can't fall asleep within 30 minutes, get up and do something else like reading, listening to music, or journaling until you feel tired. Just make sure to keep the lights low and avoid screens to support healthy circadian activity. If you find you're still awake at 3:00 a.m., consider a natural sleep aid like one of the supplements below.

Sleep Supplements

Sometimes you need a little extra help nodding off or sleeping through the night. But prescription and over-the-counter (OTC) sleep aids aren't the answer. Here's why: You can become dependent on prescription sleep aids, like Ambien or Lunesta,

and even OTC remedies, like ZzzQuil or Unisom. Prescription and OTC products can also trigger next-day grogginess, dizziness, headache, dry mouth, and digestive problems in some people. This is why I strongly recommend reaching for a natural option instead. Not only are the following supplements effective; they are also extremely safe and won't leave you feeling groggy in the morning.

Lavender. Sniffing this fragrant herb or spritzing its essential oil on your pillow before turning in has been clinically shown to naturally induce sleep. But did you know that lavender can also be taken internally as a supplement or tea to ease anxiety and foster better sleep? During one double-blind, randomized study of 77 people with generalized anxiety disorder, taking an oral lavender supplement was found to be just as effective as the anti-anxiety drug lorazepam for reducing anxiety and improving the quality of sleep. Another trial found that supplementing with lavender for six weeks also reduced the number of times the participants woke up in the middle of the night. If you'd like to try supplementing with lavender (as opposed to using it for its aromatherapeutic benefits), look for a supplement that's specifically designed to be used orally and made from oil derived exclusively from the aerial (above ground) parts of the plant.

Lemon Balm. If anxiety is keeping you up at night, consider lemon balm. With a long history of use in Europe, modern research reports that this unique botanical reduces stress and anxiety while also improving mood. In one small double-blind, placebo-controlled, crossover trial, supplementing with lemon balm effectively reduced stress. A more recent study that appeared in the Mediterranean Journal of Nutrition and Metabolism found that a lemon-balm extract not only reduced the symptoms of stress and anxiety but also improved sleep in as little as 15 days.

Mandarin. Often used in Traditional Chinese Medicine for relaxation, mandarin has been clinically shown to beneficially act on the nervous system. Findings in the journal Molecules reported that mandarin influences brain waves by decreasing alpha waves, which mimic the brain activity experienced right before you fall asleep, and by increasing theta waves, the brain waves that are active during REM and non-REM sleep. These actions give mandarin its sleep-inducing properties.

Ravintsara. Native to the Madagascar rain forest, ravintsara contains an oil in the leaves and bark that is rich in an anti-inflammatory compound, called 1,8-cineole, that has been shown to balance cognition and ease anxiety. Although you can get some sleep-supporting benefits when used as an aromatherapeutic oil, if you want to take it as a supplement, look for a supercritical CO2 extract specifically designed for oral use. You may also find it included in a sleep-specific formula that combines lemon balm, lavender, and mandarin.

Magnesium. This essential mineral plays a role in more than 300 biochemical reactions in the body—from regulating your blood glucose levels to supporting your cardiovascular health to relaxing your muscles. But magnesium also plays a key role in promoting good-quality sleep thanks to its ability to relax both body and mind. Studies show that this can help you fall asleep faster and improve your overall sleep quality. During one of these studies, older adults were given 500 mg of supplemental magnesium or a placebo each day for eight weeks. Those taking the magnesium reported falling asleep faster, sleeping longer, and waking more refreshed than those taking the placebo. Other studies suggest that a daily dose of magnesium may help to reverse some of the biological changes affecting sleep as you grow older. This is because magnesium helps regulate melatonin production. And because this mineral also binds to GABA receptors, it acts to relax the nervous system. Just be aware that some forms of supplemental magnesium can overstimulate the bowels and trigger diarrhea, especially at higher doses. That's why I always take a chelated magnesium glycinate supplement. This form is bound to the amino acid glycine, making it easily absorbed in the body and gentle on the intestinal tract.

Melatonin. This hormone-like compound is probably the most well-known supplement among those struggling to get a good night's sleep. Naturally made in the pineal gland, melatonin regulates your circadian rhythms and therefore your sleep-wake cycle. But the amount of melatonin the body makes declines with age. Fortunately, studies show that when taken as a supplement, melatonin reduces the time it takes to fall asleep, increases sleep quality, and boosts the amount of sleep you get. As a bonus, melatonin also supports healthy blood sugar levels, cholesterol levels, and immunity. But to get the full benefits melatonin provides, look for a sustained-release form, listed on product labels as EP120. I recommend taking 3 to 10 mg of melatonin as needed.

TRACKING YOUR SLEEP

Millions of people are using smartphone apps, bed monitors, and wearable items, such as smart watches or rings, to collect and analyze their sleep data. Smart technology can record sounds and movement during sleep, track the total number of hours slept, tell you how much of that time was spent in each stage of sleep, and even monitor your heart rate, body temperature, and breathing. Most wearable devices sync with your smartphone so you have all of your sleep data at your fingertips. If wearing a device while you sleep isn't your cup of tea, you can also find sleep-tracking pads that work under your mattress. This may be especially beneficial for couples looking to monitor the quality and duration of their sleep. But all of this data comes at a price. Wearable devices can range from $50 to $400. Under-mattress trackers can set you back $85 to a whopping $3,200. Despite the price, tapping into your sleep data may provide you with the intel you need to improve your sleep quality and duration. But before purchasing any sleep tracker, do your research. Check the reviews and, if possible, talk to friends and family who may have experience with the device you're considering.

CHAPTER 8

Stress Less

Stress is a fact of life. Whether it's due to work, money, or relationships, everyone experiences psychological stress at some time or other. Add in worry about the economy, global events, climate change, and other world concerns and it's no wonder more than 75 percent of Americans report feeling stressed and anxious.

• • • • • • • • • • •

But is stress always a bad thing? Not necessarily. After all, stress is the driver behind much of the progress humanity has made through the centuries. This is because short-term stress can generate the impetus necessary to convert thought into action, whether that action is escaping from a dangerous situation or simply meeting a deadline at work. But to truly understand the effect stress has on our lives, it's important to get a clear picture of what it is.

Stress: The Good, The Bad, and The Ugly

When we feel like we're in danger—whether that danger is real or simply perceived—the body experiences a complex chain of biological changes that instantly put us on alert and help ensure our survival. Known as the "fight or flight" response, this action involves the brain, the immune system, and the hypothalamus-pituitary-adrenal (HPA) axis. It all starts in the hypothalamus, a tiny cluster of cells at the base of the brain that controls all automatic body functions. The hypothalamus triggers nerve cells to release norepinephrine, a hormone that tightens the muscles and sharpens the senses. At the same time, the adrenal glands release epinephrine, better known as adrenaline, which makes the heart pump faster and the lungs work harder to flood the body with oxygen. The adrenal glands also release the hormone cortisol, which helps the body convert sugar to energy. Historically, once the threat had passed, the parasympathetic branch of the autonomic nervous system would take over, allowing the body to return to normal. But that was then, and this is now.

Unlike our ancestors, who had to deal with only the occasional saber-toothed tiger or club-wielding enemy, we are often subjected to 50 or more stressors a day. And that's a problem since our bodies can't make the distinction between the life-threatening events, like a natural disaster or mugging, and the frustration of being stuck in a traffic jam. As a result, we're stressed much of the time, and this has led to a variety of stress-related illnesses. In fact, it's estimated that 80 percent of all visits to the doctor are for stress-induced illnesses, including cardiovascular disease, diabetes, gastrointestinal problems, immunity, and neurological conditions.

Cardiovascular disease. Chronically high cortisol levels can have a negative impact on the cardiovascular system. In one long-term Swedish study of more than 136,000 people with stress-related disorders, researchers found that unrelenting stress was strongly linked to an increased risk of arrhythmia, deep vein thrombosis, and heart failure. They also noted that stress appeared to be strongly associated with developing these cardiovascular problems at an earlier age than the participants' less-stressed counterparts. Other studies have shown a connection between chronic stress and the risk of developing atherosclerosis, high blood pressure, and unhealthy cholesterol levels. Unrelenting stress also increases the risk of dying of a cardiovascular event like a heart attack or stroke.

Diabetes. Stress is also a strong risk factor for type 2 diabetes. In one study of 12,844 women taking part in the Australian Longitudinal Study on Women's Health, researchers found that those routinely dealing with moderate to high stress levels had a 2.3 times greater risk of type 2 diabetes. Other research reports that men who are chronically stressed have a 45 percent higher risk of developing the condition. According to some researchers, people suffering from chronic stress, anxiety, or anger may be at a higher risk of developing the condition because of elevated cortisol levels. They also think that these high levels might stop beta cells in the pancreas from working properly, reducing the amount of insulin made.

Gastrointestinal disorders. Persistently elevated cortisol levels can also wreak havoc with your gastrointestinal system either by delaying the emptying of the stomach or by speeding up the amount of time it takes food and waste to pass through the colon. But the negative effects of stress on your digestive tract don't stop there. Recent research out of China shows that the stress hormones cortisol, epinephrine, and norepinephrine also disrupt the bacterial balance in the gut and trigger gastrointestinal inflammation. This may, at least partially, explain why stress can cause a flare-up in those with irritable bowel syndrome or an inflammatory bowel disease.

Immunity. If you've ever gotten sick right after a stressful event, you've personally seen how stress can affect your immune system. Although the immune system is initially given a boost during the fight-or-flight response, if stress persists, the nutrients needed to support the body's physical and mental demands are depleted. Living in a world of wall-to-wall stress also results in immune-suppressing levels of the stress hormones epinephrine and norepinephrine.

And high cortisol levels can put a damper on the activity of your natural killer cells—the specialized immune cells that target viruses and other threats.

Neurological conditions. When it comes to the health of your brain, too much stress can lead to poor concentration, depression, and the uneasy feeling that you're not really in charge of your own life. The Hopi Native Americans have a name for it—koyaanisqatsi, meaning "life out of balance." Ongoing stress can trigger a steady flood of cortisol and prolonged activation of the HPA axis, significantly increasing the risk of cognitive decline. This is because long-term activation of the HPA axis targets the hippocampus, which is involved in learning and memory; the amygdala, which processes fearful emotions and memories; and the prefrontal cortex, which is the seat of cognitive function.

Over time, chronic stress can leave you increasingly vulnerable to Alzheimer's disease and other forms of dementia. According to one study out of the University of Texas Health Science Center, stress drives Alzheimer's disease by activating neural and endocrine pathways, which causes an uptick in the formation of beta-amyloid protein. This, in turn, boosts the amount of amyloid plaque in the brain—a hallmark of Alzheimer's. Preliminary research also suggests that stress accelerates the loss in cognitive function by changing the way another protein known as tau functions. Normally, tau molecules attach themselves to structures in the brain called microtubules, and they're important for maintaining healthy neurons. But long-term stress causes tau molecules to form tangles that, instead of protecting neurons, actually destroy them.

People with seizure disorders such as epilepsy also find that stress can worsen their condition and actually trigger a seizure. In one retrospective study, Dutch scientists compared the seizure activity

COMMON CAUSES OF STRESS

Stress-triggering events can weaken your immune system and, as you've seen, make you more vulnerable to a host of diseases. While just about anything can cause stress, whether real or perceived, some of the most common stressors are:

- Chronic illness or injury
- Death of a loved one
- Divorce
- Financial difficulties
- Getting married
- Losing your job
- Moving
- Pregnancy
- Retirement
- Sexual difficulties
- Taking care of an elderly or sick family member
- The birth of a child
- Work difficulties
- World events

of 30 epileptic patients suddenly evacuated because of an impending flood to 30 patients living outside the evacuation area. What they found was that one-third of the evacuees experienced a significant increase in the frequency of their seizures compared to those who had not experienced the flood-related stress.

How can you rebalance your life when stress seems to be everywhere? The secret isn't in avoiding the pressures of everyday life. It's learning to mitigate the harmful effects that come from chronic stress. Fortunately, there are a number of natural ways to create a healthy ratio of positive to negative stress.

Stress Busters

Allowing yourself to become a victim of ongoing stress not only undermines your physical health; it can also damage your mental and emotional well-being. But you can limit the harm stress causes by employing one or more of the following strategies:

Aromatherapy. Think about how you feel when you smell fresh bread as it comes out of the oven or newly cut grass. These scents likely evoke a pleasant emotional response. But aromatherapy doesn't just trigger happy memories associated with specific odors. Aromatherapy is a well-accepted holistic healing treatment that uses natural essential oils to ease stress and promote health and well-being. These essential oils comprise naturally occurring chemicals that are volatile and evaporate quickly.

Because of this, their molecules are easily inhaled, and they provide triggers to the areas of the brain that control emotions and stress response.

Although aromatherapy should not be considered a miracle cure for serious emotional issues, it can—depending on the essential oil used—lift your spirits, calm you down, or boost your energy levels. Additionally, the proper use of essential oils may help you cope with day-to-day challenges. In one study that appeared in the journal *Alternative & Integrative Medicine,* women who received an aromatherapeutic massage using a blend of lavender and chamomile essential oils reported a 12 percent drop in stress and a 30 percent reduction in feelings of anxiety compared to a placebo group. Other studies found that this same blend not only helped those experiencing stress and anxiety, it also helped relieve depression in older adults.

If you'd like to try aromatherapy, make sure to use only high-quality essential oils. These highly concentrated oils are the volatile oils from herbs, barks, and flowers, which are processed via steam distillation or expression. Avoid products labeled as essence oils, perfume oils, or fragrance oils. Look for color variations and check the label for a statement warning against its undiluted use, which indicates that you are buying a pure, therapeutic-strength essential oil.

Essential oils are generally safe to inhale or use topically. Typically, pure essential oils should be diluted with a carrier oil like almond oil since some essential oils can cause a skin reaction if used at full strength.

Never take an essential oil internally unless advised to do so by a practitioner who is qualified or licensed to prescribe essential oils in this way.

Breath work. When you are stressed, your muscles tighten and your breathing becomes quick and shallow. As you breathe more lightly, you trigger a vicious cycle because your body responds to your change in breathing with a fight-or-flight response, adding to your tension and stress. To counteract this, the most basic thing you can do when you start to feel stressed is to stop and take some deep, even, and slow breaths. There are many ways to practice breath work. Some, like qigong or yogic breathing, are best done under the guidance of an instructor. But just taking 5 or 10 deep breaths—and concentrating fully on each breath—can be tremendously helpful in soothing stressful moments.

You can also try box breathing. Practiced by Navy SEALs, this technique involves breathing deeply from your belly, which slows the breath and helps ease stress. Here's why it works: When you're stressed, your sympathetic nervous system is on high alert, and your breath moves from your belly to your chest. Box breathing takes you out of the fight-or-flight state and activates your parasympathetic nervous system. This taps into your body's rest-and-digest mode and effectively helps downgrade those feelings of stress.

The next time you're stressed out, give box breathing a try. It's really quite simple if you follow these six easy steps:

1. Slowly breathe out, expelling all the air from your lungs.

2. Breathe in through your nose as you slowly and silently count to four. Focus on how the air fills your lungs.

3. Hold your breath for a count of four.

4. Slowly exhale for another count of four.

5. Don't breathe for a count of four.

6. Repeat the entire process three or four more times.

Journaling. Sometimes the simple act of writing down what's on your mind can help foster calm. This type of "brain dump" can be helpful before turning in at night, especially if you're the type of person who tends to lie in bed with your thoughts and worries racing about. Journaling can also help clarify your feelings, giving you deeper insight into your responses to stress. Experiment with these different types of journaling to see what works best for you.

✦ **Bullet Journal.** This quick and easy way of journaling can help keep track of all the things you need to do each day, as well as your goals, aspirations, and memories. Writing things down can relieve stress by helping you unclutter your mind and prioritize the tasks for the day. Being more organized and balanced is a great way to feel less stressed and more in control.

✦ **Emotional-Release Journal.** Writing down your emotional responses to stressful events can help you process what you are feeling and perhaps allow you to reframe these events and your responses in a more positive way. To begin, purchase a blank journal and set aside time at the end of each day to write about the people or events that triggered an emotional response. Ask yourself why you're having such a strong reaction—have you always reacted this way to a particular kind of person, event, or situation? If so, what do all of these triggers have in common? Over time, you'll not only gain a better understanding of your emotional triggers and responses, but you'll also begin to find healthier ways to deal with these stressors.

✦ **Gratitude Journal.** Remembering what you're grateful for or what brings you joy can shift your mindset from your worries to appreciating the positive people and things in your life. This not only helps improve your mood in the moment; it also helps build long-term resilience for the times when stress seems to surround you. To start keeping a gratitude journal, simply write down at least three things you're grateful for every day. As a bonus, a gratitude journal also works as a record of the good things in your life that you can reflect on during the times when you're feeling down.

Laughter. Laughter is good for the soul, and recent studies indicate that using a little jocularity to manage stress can help reverse the cardiovascular-damaging effects of stress hormones. Better yet, researchers at Indiana State University have found that a good belly laugh boosts natural killer–cell activity and increases overall immune function.

Besides helping keep you physically and mentally balanced, humor can make you feel in charge of your life. After all, you can't always control the situations around you, but you can control your internal responses to them with humor. Try spending 5 or 10 minutes a day looking for the funny side of life. Create a humor bulletin board and tack up cartoons and jokes that make you chuckle. Regularly watch movies that leave you rolling on the floor. Collect silly things that make you laugh—children's toys, clown noses, funny hats—and play with them often. Or create a "mirth-aid" kit full of things that tickle your funny bone for those times when stress gets the better of you.

Massage. A host of mind-body benefits can be attributed to the age-old practice of therapeutic massage. According to the American Massage Therapy Association (AMTA), massage boosts the immune system by increasing the number of natural killer cells, which tend to break down during stress. Massage can also increase circulation, reduce muscle tension, stimulate lymphatic drainage, control musculoskeletal pain, ease migraines, increase alertness and energy levels, and boost feelings of well-being.

There are a number of different types of massage. Eastern massage focuses on balancing the body's energy flow to produce good health. One type of Japanese massage uses choreographed movements that emphasize rhythm, pacing, precision, and form. Swedish massage approaches the body from an anatomical point of view and employs gliding, stroking, and friction to soothe the body. Aromatherapeutic massage combines the best of Swedish massage with aromatherapy to ease anxiety and fatigue. Whichever type of massage you choose, the AMTA advises finding a certified therapist. To help you locate one in your area, the AMTA maintains a database of qualified massage therapists on their website, *amtamassage.org/find-massage-therapist*. To get the most from massage therapy, plan on visiting your masseuse at least once a month since the benefits aren't sustained or cumulative.

Meditation. As more people discover the benefits of meditation, the old counterculture image of navel-gazing gurus in a cloud of incense is being replaced by mainstream portraits of people from all walks of life engaging in this ancient practice. Learning to meditate not only helps put stress in perspective; it offers real health benefits. According to the National Center for Complementary and Integrative Health, meditation reduces blood pressure, irritable bowel syndrome symptoms, anxiety and depression, and insomnia. It may also ease pain and help people deal with the emotions and stress that surrounds conditions like cancer, heart disease, and menopause.

In one study of 93 people with generalized anxiety disorder, researchers from the Department of Psychiatry at Massachusetts General Hospital found that those who practiced a type of meditation known as mindfulness meditation felt less anxious and, over time, experienced an improvement in the way they react to stress. Another study, this time involving pharmacy students, found that regular meditation practice minimized the feelings of stress and improved overall mental well-being.

There are several different types of meditation, including mindfulness meditation, concentrative meditation, and transcendental meditation. In mindfulness meditation, practitioners simply witness whatever goes through their minds without reacting or becoming involved with those thoughts or worries. Concentrative meditation focuses on something tangible—an image or a sound—in order to still the mind and allow a greater awareness to emerge. In both forms, meditators become keenly aware of their reactions to stress, allowing them to gain a better sense of control over their lives.

Transcendental meditation (TM) is perhaps the most-studied form of meditation. Practitioners strive to improve health through a twice-daily practice of controlled breathing, the repetition of a particular word or sound, called a mantra, and an emptying of the mind. One reason for this, say researchers at Reina Sofía University Hospital in Córdoba, Spain, is that the regular practice of TM has a significant effect on the sympathetic nervous system. In the study, 19 practitioners of TM were compared with 16 volunteers who had never used any type of relaxation therapy. Throughout the study, the researchers measured the amounts of norepinephrine and epinephrine in the participants' blood and found that those practicing TM had consistently lower plasma levels of these stress hormones. Other studies have found that adopting a regular TM practice effectively reduces cortisol levels by as much as 30 percent.

One of the easiest ways to start meditating is with a smart phone–based app like Calm or Headspace. These apps, which are available for both iOS and android devices, provide guided meditation for a variety of situations and can be customized to specific topics or amounts of time.

Music. No doubt you've heard the old adage that "music has charms to soothe a savage breast." And it's true. But music doesn't just have the ability to reduce stress. It can also promote healing and improve your overall well-being. Research demonstrates that listening to music in addition to standard therapy is more effective than therapy alone for people with anxiety and depression. Other studies have found that music can ease stress and anxiety in critically ill people. Even simply listening to relaxing music throughout the day can reduce feelings of stress. Ditto for those who enjoy playing an instrument or singing along to their favorite songs.

Why does music have such a calming effect on our stress levels? Studies show that music stimulates the production of dopamine, that feel-good neurotransmitter in the brain. In fact, when a group of Canadian researchers examined images of patients who listened to music while undergoing an MRI, they were able to see a dopamine boost in the same areas of the brain associated with pleasure.

Listening to music is so effective that it might even help prevent burnout. This was shown in a study of frontline nurses who experience stress on the job every day. During the study, which appeared in the *Journal of Advanced Nursing,* the nurses who listened to relaxing music for 30 minutes during their break had lower perceived-stress levels, lower cortisol levels, and lower heart rates than the nurses who didn't listen to music. So the next time stress threatens to overwhelm your day, spend a few minutes listening to your favorite playlist. It just might help brighten your mood!

Prayer. Studies show that prayer can help alleviate stress and improve coping skills. This makes sense since prayer helps you "hand over" stressful feelings or worry to a greater power. This was shown in a study of more than 1,200 medical professionals. The participants reported that prayer improved their ability to cope with on-the-job stress and fostered a greater sense of calm. According to author and minister Max Lucado, when you're stressed it's important to pray immediately instead of letting unsettling thoughts swirl in your brain. He also recommends being specific as you pray, praying for and with others when possible, and bringing gratitude into your prayer practice. As he notes, anxiety and gratitude cannot occupy the same space in the brain. When you catalog what you are thankful for, your list of challenges grows less powerful.

Progressive muscle relaxation. Progressive muscle relaxation is a popular stress-busting technique first introduced in the 1930s by American physician Edmund Jacobson. It involves tightening and then relaxing all of the body's major muscle groups, beginning at the head and ending with the toes. Studies have found that practicing progressive muscle relaxation—especially while listening to some relaxing music—effectively reduces stress and fatigue while also improving coping skills.

To practice progressive muscle relaxation, find a quiet place free from any distractions. Lie on the floor or your bed, or sit in a comfortable chair and take a few deep breaths from your diaphragm. To begin, focus your attention on each of the following areas, one at a time:

1. **Forehead:** Tighten the muscles in your forehead and hold for 15 seconds. Then slowly release the tension while counting to 30 and breathing slowly and evenly.

2. **Neck and shoulders:** Increase the tension in your neck and shoulders by raising your shoulders up toward your ears. Hold for 15 seconds, then slowly release the tension for another count of 30.

3. **Arms and hands:** Make a fist with each hand, then slowly draw them into your chest. Hold for 15 seconds, squeezing as tightly as you can. Gradually open your hands as you slowly lower them to your sides to a count of 30.

4. **Buttocks:** Gradually tense the muscles in your buttocks over 15 seconds. Then slowly release the tension over 30 seconds. Continue to breathe slowly and evenly.

5. **Legs:** Slowly squeeze the muscles in your quadriceps and calves and hold for 15 seconds. Gently release the tension as you count to 30.

6. **Feet:** Focus on your feet and gradually increase the tension in the arches and toes. Slowly release the tension while you count to 30.

Yoga. This mind-body practice consists of a series of asanas, or poses, combined with a specific way of breathing that reduces stress, improves mental function, and exercises the body. There are many different styles of yoga, such as Bikram, Iyengar, and Kundalini. But when it comes to stress, Hatha yoga may be just what the doctor ordered. Hatha yoga is slower, and beginners find the asanas easier than those common to other forms. It's also been shown to be highly effective for lowering stress. According to findings in the International Journal of Preventive Medicine, women who participated in 12 Hatha yoga sessions reported a significant decrease in anxiety, depression, and stress. Even a single yoga session can provide calming benefits. This was shown in a 2013 study, which found that just one 90-minute yoga class significantly eased feelings of perceived stress in middle-aged women.

Since yoga can be adapted for any number of circumstances, you can take up the practice no matter your age or fitness level. Classes can be found in most cities across America. If you'd rather develop a home-based practice, you can tap into a variety of YouTube videos that can help you discover your inner Zen.

Herbal Help

While the relaxation techniques above can improve your stress response, sometimes you need a little extra help. When my life becomes a bit too stressful, I turn to echinacea. I know what you're thinking—echinacea is an immune-boosting herb that's popular during cold and flu season. But, although studies do show that one type of echinacea, known as *Echinacea purpurea*, can help fight off colds and infections, there's another specialized root extract of a specific type of echinacea, known as *Echinacea angustifolia,* that can actually foster calm.

During a recent clinical trial, researchers at the Institute of Experimental Medicine in Budapest, Hungary, found that this specialized form of echinacea significantly reduced stress and anxiety—and it did so quickly. The trial, which was published in *Phytotherapy Research,* found that healthy but stressed-out people who took 40 mg of the herb experienced a significant reduction in their anxiety within just three days. Better yet, standardized anxiety testing with the State-Trait Anxiety Inventory test showed that the calming effects of the herb persisted during the two weeks that followed the seven-day study. And the herb was well tolerated with no adverse effects like drowsiness or addiction common to some pharmaceutical anti-anxiety drugs. To experience these benefits for yourself, check the label for *Echinacea angustifolia*

root extract EP107, which is standardized for proprietary echinacosides.

Adapt with Adaptogens

Adaptogenic herbs can also help your body resist the negative effects of stress. Topping the list is the Ayurvedic herb ashwagandha. In one prospective, randomized, double-blind, placebo-controlled study, the stress-relieving effects of Ashwagandha root extract were investigated in 60 stressed but otherwise healthy adults. After eight weeks, those taking the herb experienced less perceived stress and significantly better sleep. They also had lower cortisol levels. A more recent trial found that ashwagandha works directly with the HPA axis, reducing its activity to counteract the negative aspects of stress. Some research suggests that ashwagandha also influences GABA and serotonin activity. GABA, or gamma-aminobutyric acid, is a neurotransmitter that blocks the impulses between nerve cells in the brain. Serotonin, on the other hand, is a neurotransmitter that helps regulate mood, digestion, and sleep. Low levels of either of these brain chemicals have been linked to anxiety and poor coping skills.

Be aware, however, that not every ashwagandha supplement is equally effective. The secret sauce to ashwagandha's anti-stress benefits is a compound called withanolide. Yet, studies show that because some ashwagandha supplements aren't readily absorbed and utilized by the body, the withanolides they contain can't fully interact with the HPA axis. When stress looms large, I turn to a concentrated form of ashwagandha listed on supplement labels as EP35. This proprietary form is created using the leaves and roots of the herb, and it provides seven times more withanolides than ordinary ashwagandha supplements.

Another highly effective adaptogen is rhodiola. Research indicates that rhodiola increases the body's resistance to stress, reduces fatigue, improves memory, enhances concentration and physical fitness, and increases overall well-being. If that weren't impressive enough, other studies show that rhodiola stimulates the immune system, enabling the body's own defenses to further ward off the effects of stress.

According to a recent study in *Frontiers in Pharmacology,* rhodiola may accomplish all of these tasks thanks to its antioxidant and anti-inflammatory properties and its ability to improve blood flow and metabolism in the brain. Remember that for any herbal product, the source matters. Check the label to ensure your supplement is standardized to contain more than 3% rosavins and 1% salidroside for best results.

While these tools won't eliminate stress, using them on a regular basis can help you cope with life's daily hassles and make your body less responsive to the stress hormones that can lead to disease. The reward is a healthier, happier life.

STRESS AND THE GUT-BRAIN AXIS

Stress doesn't just happen in your brain. It may actually begin in your gut. Emerging science, dubbed psychobiotics, suggests that the gut and the brain "talk" to each other via the body's longest cranial nerve—the vagus nerve. A host of new studies has discovered that the bacteria in your gut are constantly sending messages to your brain that help regulate your mood, behavior, and cognition. This is why it's critical to support a healthy microbiome. And one easy way to do that is to add a daily serving of fermented foods, such as goat's milk yogurt, kefir, kimchi, kombucha, or sauerkraut, to the recommendations found in Chapter 4. It's also smart to take a daily probiotic.

CHAPTER 9

Add Supplements

If you've already incorporated many of the dietary and lifestyle changes I've discussed so far in this book, congratulations! You're well on your way to improving your health and well-being. Yet it can be hard for most to eat perfectly, exercise, and practice healthy habits 24/7. Fortunately, dietary supplements can fill in any nutritional gaps and bolster your resiliency so you can better deal with the numerous slings and arrows that modern life throws at you.

• • • • • • • • • •

Yet, as valuable as these add-on nutrients can be, the world of supplements can be fraught with confusion. Think about it—when you walk into a health-food store, you're typically faced with row upon row of shelves filled with supplements. What's good? What works? What's backed by science? Let's face it: knowing which supplements provide the nutrients you need is often hard. But here's the good news: you don't need an advanced degree in physiology or nutrition to identify the

supplements that can help optimize your health. I'll show you exactly what you need to know!

Quality Counts

Before we get into how specific supplements can support a healthy lifestyle, let's take a moment to talk about quality. When it comes to buying clothes or a piece of furniture, it's easy to spot a high-quality product by looking for superior materials and good workmanship. However, when you're in the market for a supplement, it can be exceptionally hard to uncover quality by simply looking at the label—and that's especially true if you just rely on the label located on the front of the bottle or package. This is because, along with listing the name of the supplement, the number of capsules, softgels, or tablets the product contains, and sometimes the amount in each dose, the front label is often used for marketing claims about the product. These claims can include things like "#1 Doctor Recommended," "Advanced Formula," and "Superior Absorption." While there's typically nothing wrong with these claims, to get the full picture of what a supplement actually provides, you need to check the

Supplement Facts label found on the back of the bottle or package. According to the FDA, the Supplement Facts label must list the active ingredients, the amount per serving, and any other ingredients, such as fillers, binders, or flavorings, in the product. This gives you the basics on what's in a supplement. To get the most out of the supplements you take, however, you need more than the basics.

Because I've worked in the dietary-supplement industry for more than fifty years, I can tell you that quality and research matter. And I'm not alone. A number of supplement manufacturers set a high bar for the products they sell. These supplements are produced following strict adherence to Current Good Manufacturing Practices (CGMPs) set by the FDA.

Along with a rigorous commitment to CGMPs, responsible manufacturers ensure that every product—from the raw materials to the completed formulations—adheres to the highest standards. These standards include guaranteeing the purity of the ingredients in each supplement and making sure that ethical practices are used while harvesting or sourcing those ingredients and that each formula contains ingredients backed by credible scientific research. What's more, when purchasing a high-quality supplement, you can rest assured that the label accurately reflects what's in the bottle and that it has been manufactured, stored, and shipped in a way that maintains its efficacy and viability.

These are standards I've always adhered to when creating my Terry Naturally line

of supplements. And these are the same standards that you should insist upon when choosing a dietary supplement for your own use.

So how can you make sure these standards are met? Do your homework! Once you know how to correctly decipher a Supplement Facts label, it's wise to investigate the company that produces a supplement you're considering. Don't go with a supplement just because it has a pretty label or flashy marketing. And don't buy the cheapest supplement on the shelf. Quality costs. And investing in a high-quality supplement now may just save you thousands in health-related costs later. Bottom line? Don't settle for less than the best.

The Core Four

There are certain nutrients everyone needs, regardless of their health status or how careful they are about the foods they eat. Even if your shopping cart contains nothing but organic produce and grass-fed meat, you're likely missing out on some of the nutrients you need for optimal health. And it's even worse if you rely on a conventional supermarket or convenience store to sustain you.

If you remember what we discussed in Chapter 3, the foods you find in most grocery stores are often less than nutritious. For instance, the produce you buy there has likely been grown in nutrient-poor soil or subjected to agricultural chemicals that can alter the food's nutritional content. Adding insult to injury, these fruits and veggies are

HOW TO READ A SUPPLEMENT LABEL

A step-by-step guide to understanding the supplement label and the assurances of the USP Verified Mark

Look for the USP Verified Mark
USP stands for the United States Pharmacopeia, a scientific, nonprofit organization that sets federally recognized public standards of quality for medicines, dietary supplements, and foods. The USP mark means the supplement has been independently tested to confirm the product meets USP quality standards.

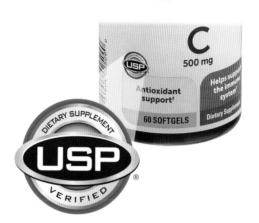

GET THE FACTS–CHECK THE BACK
The back of the label is where you will find a wealth of information. In addition to items required by law–like the manufacturer's address, lot number, or notice of potential allergens–USP verifies the label claims for accuracy and requires additional information to help you make an informed choice.

SUGGESTED USE AND SERVING SIZE
Dietary supplements are regulated as food, so the recommended amount is listed in terms of "Serving Size"–often in the form of the number of tablets or capsules to be consumed. USP tests each product for performance to ensure it will break down and release the ingredients into the body as intended.

SUPPLEMENT FACTS PANEL
The supplement label lists the individual ingredients contained in each tablet or capsule. USP tests products to positively confirm the identity and purity of each ingredient.

Supplement Facts
Serving Size 2 Gummy Vitamins
Servings Per Bottle 75

Amount Per Serving		% Daily Value
Calories	15	
Total Carbohydrate	4 g	1%†
Total Sugars	3 g	**
Includes 3 g Added Sugars		6%†
Vitamin A (as retinyl palmitate)	450 mcg RAE	50%
Vitamin C (as ascorbic acid and sodium ascorbate)	36 mg	40%
Vitamin D (as cholecalciferol)	25 mcg (1000 IU)	125%
Vitamin E (as dl-alpha-tocopheryl acetate)	15 mg	100%
Niacin (as inositol niacinate)	8 mg NE	50%
Vitamin B-6 (as pyridoxine HCl)	1.7 mg	100%
Folate	400 mcg DFE (240 mcg folic acid)	100%
Vitamin B-12 (as cyanocobalamin)	4.8 mcg	200%
Biotin	30 mcg	100%
Pantothenic acid (as calcium d-pantothenate)	3 mg	60%
Chromium (as chromium picolinate)	35 mcg	100%
Molybdenum (as molybdenum citrate)	11 mcg	24%
Sodium	10 mg	<1%
Inositol (as inositol niacinate)	1.5 mg	**
Boron (as boron citrate)	150 mcg	**

† Percent Daily Values are based on a 2,000 calorie diet.
** Daily Value not established.

Other ingredients: Glucose syrup, sugar, water, gelatin; less than 2% of: blend of oils (coconut and/or palm) with beeswax and/or carnauba wax

Caution: Consult with physician before taking this product if you are pregnant or nursing.

EXPIRES: 10/24/24

% DAILY VALUE
Where applicable, this value indicates the percent of the Recommended Dietary Intake (RDI) or Daily Reference Value (DRV) of a dietary ingredient that is in a serving of the product. USP tests each ingredient to ensure the potency–the strength or amount of the ingredient–matches what is declared on the label.

EXPIRATION DATE
USP requires participants to provide expiration date information and tests the product to ensure it will contain the claimed potency at the date specified.

CAUTIONS & WARNINGS
Where applicable, this information helps you understand who should avoid or take precautions when taking certain products. USP requires cautionary statements when appropriate as part of participation in our program.

often transported thousands of miles before they land on store shelves. Any nutrients the foods might have had when they were picked degrade with every mile.

Meat, poultry, and fish are typically raised in crowded, inhumane conditions and often pumped full of antibiotics and growth hormones. These all-to-common practices aren't good for the animals and they certainly aren't good for you.

And then there's all that ultra-processed food. Sure, cookies, chips, or frozen meals taste good, but these delicious treats aren't giving your body the information it needs for optimal health. In fact, despite claims of added vitamins and minerals splashed on food labels, these fake foods offer nothing but empty calories filled with unhealthy fats, refined sugar, and less than ideal sources of salt.

Enter supplements. Don't get me wrong —these add-on nutrients will never, ever take the place of wholesome, minimally processed foods. They can, however, help fill in the gaps caused by modern agricultural practices and food scientists only out to help farmers and food manufacturers make a buck. So let's jump into the four critical supplements everyone needs.

A Multivitamin/Multimineral

Are you getting all the necessary vitamins and minerals at the levels your body requires? As you've seen, the sad fact is that most people probably aren't. But even if your diet is textbook perfect, other factors can deplete the nutrients you need.

Topping the list is stress. Recent findings in the journal *Advances in Nutrition* report that chronic stress can drain your stores of magnesium, zinc, calcium, iron, and niacin. Other everyday factors that can leave you lacking include poor sleep; the use of certain medications like some antibiotics, blood pressure meds, and proton pump inhibitors; and inactivity.

Even if none of these factors apply to you, there's one thing you can't avoid: aging. As you grow older, your body's ability to absorb the nutrients in food declines. And studies report that this is especially true if you are among the 85 percent of people over the age of 65 with at least one chronic condition. Another problem? Older adults often eat less as they age, so by default they likely don't get the full complement of nutrients they need. But simply adding a high-quality multi can help ensure you're getting a bit of extra nutritional insurance to support good health.

What the Science Says

There's a lot of hype surrounding multivitamin/multimineral supplements. Ads often portray these supplements with images of happy people living a healthy, active life. The underlying message? This can be you—if you take our product. Don't get me wrong, I believe that taking a multi as part of a whole-body health strategy is a smart move. But if you think that simply relying on a pill can keep you healthy despite a poor diet and sedentary lifestyle—well, as Johnny Depp said in the 1997 crime drama *Donnie Brasco*, "Fuhgeddaboudit!"

That said, studies show that a multi-vitamin/multimineral can help improve health and prevent some chronic conditions. For instance, researchers evaluating 18,530 men taking part in the Physicians' Health Study found that a multi reduced the risk of needing a coronary angioplasty or coronary artery bypass graft by as much as 14 percent. And those who had taken a multi for 20 years or more also had a lower risk of heart attack or stroke. Another study found that women who took a multi for at least three years had a 44 percent lower risk of dying of heart disease.

A good-quality multi may also reduce your risk of developing some types of cancer. A 2006 study review conducted at Johns Hopkins University involving 47,289 people found that men, but not women, who took multivitamins had a 31 percent lower risk of any cancer.

Multivitamin/multimineral use has also been found to support a healthy brain. During the 2021 COSMOS mind study, which was presented at the 14th Clinical Trials on Alzheimer's Disease conference, researchers found that taking a multivitamin for three years slowed cognitive aging by as much as 60 percent. Several earlier studies also found that a multi improves memory in older adults. But a multi's mind benefits aren't just for older adults. Other research suggests that daily use may also improve cognition in young adults by helping maintain adequate levels of the B vitamins. Multivitamins might support a healthy mood by reducing the symptoms of anxiety and depression, too.

Studies also show that taking a multivitamin can support healthy vision. And that's especially true if you're at risk of cataracts or the sight-robbing condition macular degeneration. One large, ongoing study called the Age-Related Eye Disease Study (AREDS), found that a daily multi containing higher than average amounts of vitamins C and E, beta-carotene, copper, and zinc significantly slowed the progression of macular degeneration and vision loss by 27 percent. The catch? This benefit was only seen after about six years of use, meaning that you would need to supplement on a long-term basis to get results. Other studies report that the use of a multivitamin/multimineral supplement also reduces the risk of developing cataracts, a common eye condition that clouds a person's vision. One study of nearly 15,000 male physicians that appeared in the journal Ophthalmology found that long-term daily multivitamin supplementation lowered the risk of developing cataracts by as much as 13 percent.

Multivitamins can also keep you younger longer, at least at a cellular level. Research by the National Institute of Environmental Health Sciences found that women who took multivitamins had telomeres that were more than five percent longer than those who didn't supplement. Telomeres are bits of DNA located on the end of a chromosome that may play a role in how quickly cells age—so when it comes to cellular aging, longer is always better.

What to Look for in a Multi

Taking a comprehensive multivitamin/multimineral supplement provides an easy way to get the needed nutrients that you're not getting from your food. But many multis don't provide the nutrients you need in meaningful amounts. This is especially true for one-a-day formulas and gummy vitamins. And speaking of gummies, they're also often chock full of sugar and other additives that are less than healthy.

I recommend taking a comprehensive multivitamin/multimineral supplement that requires two to three doses daily. This will provide you with a steady stream of nutrients that help support all of your bodily systems. It's also important to make sure the nutrients in your supplement are in a form your body can use. To make choosing the best supplement a bit easier, I've created the following chart of the nutrients that you should look for in your multivitamin/multimineral:

WHAT TO LOOK FOR IN A MULTIVITAMIN/MULTIMINERAL SUPPLEMENT		
NUTRIENT	**BIOAVAILABLE/ACTIVE FORM**	**MINIMUM DAILY AMOUNT**
Vitamin A	Retinyl palmitate	750 mcg
Vitamin C	Calcium ascorbate	62.5 mg
Vitamin D3	Cholecalciferol	500 IU
Vitamin E	D-alpha and mixed tocopherols	250 IU
Vitamin K2	Menaquinone-7	22.5 mcg
Vitamin B2	Riboflavin	25 mg
Vitamin B3 (Niacin)	Niacinamide	25 mg
Vitamin B6	Pyridoxal 5'-phosphate	12.5 mg
Folate	Calcium L-5-methyltetrahydrofolate	340 mcg DFE
Vitamin B12	Methylcobalamin	125 mcg
Biotin	D-biotin	250 mcg
Pantothenic acid	D-calcium pantothenate	25 mcg
Choline	Choline bitartrate	25 mg
Calcium	Calcium glycinate chelate	200 mg
Iodine	Potassium iodine	75 mcg

NUTRIENT	BIOAVAILABLE/ACTIVE FORM	MINIMUM DAILY AMOUNT
Magnesium	Magnesium bisglycinate chelate	150 mg
Zinc	Zinc bisglycinate	7.5 mg
Selenium	*Saccharomyces cerevisiae*	50 mcg
Copper	Copper bisglycinate chelate	0.5 mg
Manganese	Manganese bisglycinate chelate	2.5 mg
Chromium	Chromium nicotinate glycinate chelate	125 mcg
Molybdenum	Molybdenum glycinate chelate	62.5 mcg
Potassium	Potassium glycinate chelate	25 mg
Benfotiamine	N/A	25 mg
Inositol	N/A	25 mg
Bioflavonoids	Citrus peel extract	25 mg
PABA	Para-aminobenzoic acid	7.5 mg
Boron	Calcium fructoborate	**
Vanadium	Vanadium nicotinate glycinate chelate	62.5 mcg

YOU DEFINITELY NEED A MULTI IF...

While everyone can benefit from taking a multi, some people are at particular risk for nutrient deficiencies. Factors that can increase the need for supplemental nutrients include:

- Certain medications like diuretics or proton pump inhibitors

- Malabsorption due to alcoholism, celiac disease or ulcerative colitis, or gastric bypass surgery or a Whipple procedure

- Older age, since nutrient absorption can decrease with age

- Pregnancy, since the development of a fetus increases nutrient needs in the mother

- Veganism and vegetarianism, which may not provide certain nutrients, such as vitamin B12, calcium, iron, or omega-3 fatty acids

WHY CHELATION MATTERS

You may notice that some of the minerals listed in the chart above are "chelated." Chelation is the process of transforming a mineral into a form that can be easily absorbed and used by the body. Normally, this process happens naturally in the gastrointestinal tract. The problem is, many people's natural ability to chelate minerals doesn't always work well. What's more, certain compounds, like the oxalates in spinach or the phytic acid in nuts, seeds, and grains, can decrease absorption by chemically binding to the mineral and preventing it from entering the bloodstream. Luckily, high-quality multivitamin/multimineral supplements often include minerals that have already been chelated. How can you spot them? Look for the TRAACS designation, which is a proprietary technology that chelates a mineral so your body doesn't have to.

Curcumin

A few years ago, turmeric hit fad status. From turmeric teas and "shots" to golden milk lattes, this warming Ayurvedic spice definitely had a moment. But, as popular as it was, the trendy turmeric craze didn't really live up to its healthy halo. That's because the real secret to turmeric's health benefits doesn't come from the spice itself but from a pigmented compound in the root called curcumin.

Curcumin's biggest claim to fame is its powerful anti-inflammatory capabilities. Studies show that curcumin keeps inflammation in check by downregulating the COX-2 enzyme in much the same way that aspirin or ibuprofen does. It also inhibits the metabolism of a pro-inflammatory omega-6 fatty acid called arachidonic acid, promotes apoptosis, and prevents the production of certain pro-inflammatory cytokines. It does such a good job that studies have found that curcumin is just as effective as some anti-inflammatory medications but without the adverse side effects common to many prescription drugs.

This golden compound also acts as an antioxidant, neutralizing free radicals that can lead to cellular damage. What's more, preliminary research suggests that curcumin can also boost the activity of glutathione and superoxide dismutase (SOD), two of the body's most powerful antioxidants.

Taken together, curcumin's one-two punch against inflammation and free-radical damage can prevent or benefit a surprising number of conditions:

✦ Alzheimer's disease/dementia

✦ Arthritis

✦ Cardiovascular disease

✦ Depression

✦ Inflammatory bowel disease

✦ Irritable bowel syndrome

✦ Obesity

✦ Pain

✦ Psoriasis

✦ Cancer risk

✦ Type 2 diabetes

✦ Wound healing

What the Science Says

With curcumin's ability to improve all of these conditions, it's no wonder I'm such a huge fan. In fact, because I consider it an all-in-one solution for good health, I not only take it every day, but I also think it's an essential supplement for everyone. Still think curcumin sounds too good to be true? Let's take a look at the evidence.

Studies show that curcumin promotes the development of new neurons in certain areas of the brain by boosting an important growth hormone called brain-derived neurotrophic factor, or BDNF. BDNF plays a key role in how well we age and how well we learn and perform mentally.

What's more, a 2018 study conducted at the University of California, Los Angeles, found that taking 90 mg of curcumin twice per day for 18 months improved memory by as much as 28 percent in older people suffering from mild memory loss. The curcumin also improved focus and mood. But the most exciting finding was that, when the participants underwent PET scans of their brains, those taking the curcumin had significantly less accumulation of beta-amyloid plaque and fewer tau tangles, which are two distinct signs of Alzheimer's disease.

But the brain benefits keep on coming. Other research suggests that curcumin may decrease the amount of existing beta-amyloid plaque, slow the degradation of neurons, and protect against heavy-metal toxicity. Not only can these actions benefit those with Alzheimer's or other forms of dementia; they might also help to preserve brain function in healthy adults.

Curcumin also provides mood-boosting benefits by increasing serotonin and dopamine levels in the brain. One six-week clinical trial involving 60 patients with major depression found that curcumin was just as effective for reducing symptoms as the popular antidepressant drug Prozac.

Studies also confirm curcumin's capabilities beyond the brain. Emerging clinical research suggests that the compound can lower insulin levels by as much as 26 percent. That's great news for anyone suffering from a metabolic disease like insulin resistance or type 2 diabetes. But it's also good news for the rest of us since frequent postmeal blood sugar spikes can weaken the body's immune response, contribute to eye and kidney damage, and increase the risk of a heart attack or stroke.

And speaking of the heart, curcumin's powerful antioxidant and anti-inflammatory properties also improve several all-too-common cardiovascular risk factors. First, it's been shown to prevent the artery-damaging oxidation of LDL cholesterol and lower total LDL levels. Other preclinical studies suggest that curcumin reduces triglyceride levels by as much as 27 percent and that it may play a role in preventing an enlarged heart, heart failure, and ventricular arrhythmia. One 12-week study of older adults published in the journal *Aging* found that curcumin also improved artery function by increasing the bioavailability of nitric oxide, a natural compound that dilates arteries, and by reducing oxidative stress. Another study in the *American Journal of Cardiology* found that patients who took a high dose (4,000 mg) of curcumin before and after undergoing coronary bypass surgery had a 65 percent lower risk of experiencing a heart attack while they were in the hospital.

Curcumin also reduces many types of pain thanks to its anti-inflammatory action. This can be especially beneficial for those suffering from osteoarthritis or other types of joint pain. For instance, one clinical trial of people with osteoarthritis (OA) of the knee found that curcumin reduced pain just as effectively as the prescription drug diclofenac. Further clinical study found that pairing curcumin with boswellia, another anti-inflammatory herbal compound, not only eased joint pain in OA patients but also improved morning stiffness, physical function limitations, and global assessment of disease severity scores. But curcumin doesn't just reduce joint pain. It actually protects chondrocytes—the specialized cells that make up joint cartilage—from breaking down.

The Issue of Absorption

Despite all of its benefits, curcumin does have one problem. It's not readily absorbed by the body. Whatever curcumin is absorbed is quickly metabolized and excreted from the body before it can do much good. In an attempt to increase absorption, some manufacturers use a curcumin that's combined with a black pepper extract known as piperine. Does it work to raise curcumin levels? Yes. But there's a caveat with this method—and it's kind of a big one. You see, piperine also interferes with the genes involved in your liver's ability to detoxify and eliminate drugs and toxins. What's more, piperine has been linked to the development of leaky gut.

Fortunately, I've found another form of curcumin that's been specially formulated and clinically proven to provide maximum absorption *and* bioavailability in a way that's both safe and effective. Listed on Supplement Facts labels as BCM-95, this special type of curcumin is made by combining curcumin with turmeric essential oil that's been enriched to 45 percent ar-turmerones—another active compound in turmeric. As a result, research in the *Indian Journal of Pharmaceutical Sciences* shows that BCM-95 is nearly 700 percent more bioavailable than normal curcumin supplements. It's also about six times more absorbable than supplements containing a curcumin-lecithin-piperine formula. And unlike formulas containing the black pepper extract, it won't interfere with your liver or damage your gut. I believe in the efficacy of BCM-95 so strongly that I don't just use it in the curcumin supplements I manufacture, I also take it every day without fail.

Omega-3 Fatty Acids

Even though fats often get bad-mouthed, there's one particular type of fat that's critical to good health: omega-3 fatty acids.

These fats are considered essential because the body can't make them. Instead, you must obtain them either from the foods you eat or from supplements.

There are three types of omega-3 fatty acids: docosahexaenoic acid (DHA), eicosapentaenoic acid (EPA), and alpha-linolenic acid (ALA). DHA and EPA can be found in certain types of fatty fish, such as anchovies, herring, mackerel, salmon, sardines, sea bass, trout, and tuna. ALA, on the other hand, comes from plant sources like chia seeds, flaxseeds, hemp seeds, kidney beans, seaweed, soybeans, and walnuts. But, even though vegetarians swear that ALA is a great source of omega-3s because it can be converted by the body into DHA and EPA, this conversion isn't a terribly efficient process. In fact, less than 15 percent of the ALA you eat is actually converted to DHA and EPA!

What the Science Says

So what makes omega-3s so special? Because they are so good at reducing inflammation, they can provide a number of health benefits. One 2018 study published in the *British Medical Journal* linked higher omega-3 levels with healthier aging. But that's just one benefit, albeit a pretty important one, these healthy fats provide. Studies report that omega-3s help fight the symptoms of anxiety and depression as well—and they may be just as effective as the prescription antidepressant drug Prozac.

Other research shows that omega-3s can reduce the risk of sight-robbing macular degeneration, arthritis, asthma, fatty liver disease, metabolic syndrome, osteoporosis, PMS, sarcopenia (age-related muscle loss), and more. But perhaps the most well-known benefits are centered around omega-3s impact on brain and heart health. Because omega-3s are vital to building brain and nerve cells while supporting healthy blood flow in the brain, they are critical for preserving memory and the ability to learn and reason. As a result, studies suggest that maintaining adequate omega-3 levels may help lower the risk of developing Alzheimer's disease and vascular dementia.

There's even more evidence for the wide-ranging role omega-3s play in supporting cardiovascular health. Clinical trials have found that omega-3 fatty acids boost beneficial HDL cholesterol levels while reducing triglycerides by as much as 30 percent. They have also been shown to protect the inner lining of arteries, enhance blood flow, and lower diastolic blood pressure. But the most exciting news came out of a 2021 analysis of 38 clinical trials that involved more than 149,000 people. The study review found that taking an omega-3 supplement reduced the risk of heart attack, blood clots, and the need to restore blood flow to a blocked artery, technically known as revascularization.

With all of these whole-body benefits, you can see why it's important to boost your omega-3 levels. But, while it's ideal to get DHA and EPA from fish, the truth is Americans simply don't eat enough of it. According to a 2021 study, 68 percent of adults and a whopping 95 percent of children don't get enough omega-3s from their diets to meet their nutritional needs. That's why it's so important to take an omega-3 supplement.

What to Look for

Like curcumin and multivitamins, the quality and effectiveness of omega-3 supplements can vary widely. For one thing, most supplements use fish oil that's derived from less than optimal sources like anchovies or sardines. But you'll never know because these products don't tell you where their fish oil comes from. Worse still, it's not unusual for the fish oil used in a supplement to be subjected to high heat and chemical solvents during the extraction and manufacturing process. This kind of processing damages the structure of the omega-3s and reduces their bioavailability.

Making matters even worse, fish oil supplements can become rancid as they sit on warehouse or store shelves. Rancidity arises when a product becomes oxidized—and that can make your supplement less effective and possibly even harmful. Unfortunately, rancidity is rampant. Independent testing found that, on average, 20 percent of the popular brands evaluated were rancid. A sign your fish oil isn't up to snuff? It can have a strong fishy taste and a rotten smell.

I prefer to get my omega-3s from a supplement sourced from wild salmon that's been naturally bound to phospholipids and bioactive peptides. It's much closer to the natural form of omega-3s that you'd get from eating fish. Not only does this form provide more benefit because it's

EATING YOUR OMEGAS? WHY RATIO MATTERS

Omega-3s aren't the only type of essential fatty acid. There's another one that's much more common—omega 6s. Found primarily in seed and vegetable oils, such as canola, corn, and safflower oils, omega-6s have the opposite effect than that of omega-3s in the body. Omega-6s actually stoke the fires of inflammation. And if you're eating the typical Western diet, you're getting plenty of them! Although our ancestors typically ate a ratio of 1 omega-6 to 1 omega-3, most modern Americans consume a ratio closer to 20:1, omega-6s to omega-3s. It's a ratio that's driving disease and shortening people's lives.

The good news is that you can rein in this ratio. Studies show that trading seed oils for avocado oil, coconut oil, or extra-virgin olive oil, and swapping out conventional meat for omega-3-rich wild-caught fish and grass-fed beef can provide a considerably healthier balance of omega fatty acids. What's both optimal and achievable? Shooting for a 1:1 ratio is pretty unrealistic in today's world. But according to one French study of heart attack patients, achieving a 4:1 ratio of omega-6s to omega-3s is not only possible; it can decrease total mortality by up to 70 percent.

easier for the body to utilize; you also won't experience those fishy burps standard fish oil supplements are famous for. Plus, the omega-3s in this type of supplement are stable so rancidity isn't an issue. Next time you're in the market for an omega-3 supplement, check the label for a salmon source with phospholipids and peptides to make sure you're actually getting the benefits you pay for.

Probiotics

Are you familiar with your microbiome? If not, it's high time you were introduced. Your microbiome is located primarily in your large intestine, and to a lesser degree in your small intestine, and it's home to approximately 39 trillion different microbes. This includes bacteria, viruses, and fungi, known collectively as your microbiota. But, while this might sound scary, don't panic. Most of these microbes are good guys that help keep you healthy. Together, the microbes in your gut microbiome help control the storage of fat, activate nutrient-absorbing genes, and break down toxins.

Although mankind has been aware of the microbiome for centuries, earnest studies into its role in human health didn't occur until the early 2000s. Once they did, research exploded. Not only have recent studies shown that the state of your microbiome is involved with the state of your digestive health. These investigations also discovered that your gut microbiome is intimately involved in the health of your immune system, your cardiovascular

system, and even your brain! And that's why it's absolutely vital that you do everything in your power to keep the microbiota in your microbiome well balanced and in top form.

The problem is, a number of common factors can disrupt a healthy microbial balance. These include a diet packed with ultra-processed foods high in food additives and sugar, alcohol overindulgence, smoking, antibiotic use, poor dental hygiene, sedentary living, high stress levels, and pesticide exposure. And that means a daily probiotic supplement is essential.

What the Science Says

A growing number of studies confirm that a healthy microbiome translates to whole-body health. While there are a number of beneficial probiotic strains that support good health, three are especially important: *Lactobacillus plantarum*, *Lactobacillus rhamnosus*, and *Bifidobacterium bifidum*.

L. plantarum is one of the hardiest strains of probiotics, and it's capable of surviving the journey through the harsh environment of your gastrointestinal tract. What's even more impressive is that it can even survive some antibiotics—a feat that most strains of beneficial bacteria can't accomplish. Research confirms that *L. plantarum* prevents harmful pathogens from taking hold in the gut by triggering an immune response. For instance, studies show that this powerful strain prevents or improves antibiotic-associated diarrhea and traveler's diarrhea. It's also been found to alleviate some symptoms of irritable bowel syndrome (IBS).

Beyond *L. plantarum*'s gut benefits, the strain has also been shown to reduce total cholesterol levels by as much as 13.6 percent. And in one study of postmenopausal women with metabolic syndrome, *L. plantarum* improved homocysteine blood levels. As a bonus, studies also suggest that this strain may help turn back the clock on your complexion, from the inside out. Human trials report that *L. plantarum* boosts skin hydration, improves elasticity, and reduces the depth of wrinkles for younger-looking skin.

Lactobacillus rhamnosus is another probiotic with powerful benefits. Like *L. plantarum*, it helps prevent and treat various types of diarrhea and IBS symptoms. But this particular probiotic also provides some unique benefits. For instance, during a study conducted at the University of Helsinki, Finnish researchers found that children who were given milk laced with *L. rhamnosus* most days of the week had fewer cavities than children drinking regular milk. Other studies report that consuming a probiotic containing *L. rhamnosus* significantly reduced bacterial growth and gum inflammation compared to a placebo.

In one analysis of five studies involving nearly 300 women, a probiotic containing *L. rhamnosus* also helped prevent urinary tract infections (UTIs). Other preliminary studies suggest that this potent member of the *Lactobacillus* family may increase insulin sensitivity, reduce cholesterol levels, and even prevent or improve allergy symptoms.

Bifidobacterium bifidum belongs to a different genus of beneficial bacteria. But like the two *Lactobacillus* probiotics discussed above, *B. bifidum* also supports healthy digestion and has been shown to reduce the symptoms of IBS. In one small clinical trial of IBS patients, supplementing with *B. bifidum* reduced abdominal pain, diarrhea, constipation, and dyspepsia while also improving the feelings of anger and hostility. Another trial—this one involving more than 300 people—found that this particular probiotic eased gastric and lower abdominal discomfort, as well.

Research shows that *B. bifidum* also strengthens immunity either by recruiting white blood cells to fight off an infection or by keeping inflammation in check. In one Austrian study of trained athletes, researchers at the Medical University of Innsbruck found that a daily dose of a probiotic containing *B. bifidum* prevented upper respiratory infections. Other research suggests that this strain also improves diabetic markers, including fasting blood glucose, HbA1c, and cholesterol levels, as well as insulin sensitivity.

Together, these three probiotic strains provide wide-ranging benefits that help support optimal health. No wonder a good probiotic supplement is on my must-have list.

What to Look for

Along with adopting healthier habits and feeding your gut microbiome the fiber-rich foods it craves (think veggies), one of the easiest ways to foster microbial balance is with a probiotic supplement. But choosing the right probiotics can be fraught with confusion. So many probiotic supplements!

So many different strains! And what the heck are CFUs?

First things first. Colony-forming units, or CFUs, are simply a measurement of the number of live bacterial cultures in a probiotic supplement. Research suggests that a minimum of 1 to 2 billion CFUs are needed to maintain good health. But if you're like most people and you don't eat an optimal diet 365 days a year, have taken antibiotics, have digestive problems, or suffer from Candida or frequent urinary tract infections, you'll want to boost that amount. Studies show that adults can safely take 20 billion CFUs of supplemental probiotics. Those with conditions like IBS, eczema, or weakened immune function may need even more. But no matter how much you take, it's important to take your probiotic supplement just before eating a meal that contains some fat for best absorption.

It's also important to make sure your probiotic contains the three specific strains discussed above. Although some supplements contain an astounding number of strains, not all may be beneficial for you. *L. plantarum*, *L. rhamnosus*, and *B. bifidum*, however, have been clinically shown to benefit human health, so choosing a probiotic containing these strains is a great way to support your overall health.

Additional Supplements for Specific Needs

The "core four" supplements discussed above are critical for supporting good health. But I would be remiss if I didn't mention a few other nutrients that many Americans are often low on. Adding these to your daily regimen can truly take your health to the next level.

Magnesium. This mineral is involved in more than 300 reactions in the body, ranging from energy production to healthy cholesterol balance to proper muscle and nerve function. Although magnesium is found in deep-green leafy vegetables, nuts, seeds, and dark chocolate, cooking and processing destroys this important mineral. Alcohol, coffee, and sugar can also deplete levels in the body. As a result, the National Academy of Sciences reports that 80 percent of American men and 70 percent of American women have less than adequate levels. This deficiency can have some pretty dire consequences because adequate magnesium levels are essential for healthy blood sugar levels, bone metabolism, cardiovascular health, exercise performance, pregnancy, insulin sensitivity, mood, muscle function, sleep, and stress management.

Getting enough magnesium on a daily basis requires supplementation. But if you go shopping for a magnesium supplement, be aware that there are at least 11 different forms. Some, like magnesium oxide, are cheap and essentially unusable by the body. Don't waste your money! Many other forms of magnesium, including carbonate, chloride, and gluconate, can cause diarrhea—and who needs that? My preferred form is magnesium bisglycinate chelate. Not only is this form well absorbed and utilized by the body, but it won't cause diarrhea. It's also extremely safe at doses up to 400 mg per day since any excess not used by the body is typically eliminated by the kidneys.

Vitamin D. If you live in a northern climate with limited sunlight for part of the year, spend most of your time indoors, or are a big fan of sunscreen, you're probably low on vitamin D. And that matters since this hormone-like nutrient is essential for a robust immune response, mental well-being, and a healthy weight. Low levels have been linked to autoimmune issues, cavities and gum disease, cardiovascular problems, higher risk of infection, increased odds of fractures, neurological disorders, several types of cancer, and type 2 diabetes. According to many medical experts, *everyone* should take a vitamin D supplement. I couldn't agree more. Just check the label to make sure you're getting vitamin D3, the active form your body can use.

Before taking supplemental D, have your current levels measured by a lab. Using that as a baseline, the goal is to bring your blood level up to at least a 25(OH)D concentration. This may require doses that range anywhere from 2,000 to 10,000 IU daily. For most people though, a supplement that provides 5,000 IU will do the trick.

Vitamin K2. This fat-soluble nutrient often flies under the radar—and that's a shame. Even if you have heard of vitamin K, you're likely not getting the form you need. The confusion arises because there are actually two forms of vitamin K: K1 and K2. Vitamin K1 can be found in leafy greens, and it's essential for proper blood clotting. The best sources of K2, on the other hand, come from organ meats and a Japanese fermented soy dish called natto—foods rarely, if ever, eaten in America. This is problematic since, along with proper blood clotting, K2 helps regulate cell growth, control calcium metabolism, manage vitamin D, maintain healthy blood sugar levels, and support bone, brain, and heart health.

Because it's harder to get sufficient amounts of K2 from food, it's important to supplement. But before you grab any old K2 supplement, check the label. Supplements typically provide K2 as one of two subtypes—MK-4 (menaquinone-4) and MK-7 (menaquinone-7). What's the difference? MK-4 has a shorter half-life, which means it doesn't last as long as MK-7 does in the body. Because, according to one 2019 review, the body absorbs 10 times more vitamin K2 in the form of MK-7, so make sure this is the form you're taking. How much do you need? An effective dose for most people is 180 mcg per day. But like other fat-soluble vitamins, K2 should be taken with a meal that contains some fat so you'll increase absorption even more.

Regain Your Health at Any Age!

CHAPTER 10

Optimize Your Diet

As you've learned, exercise, sleep, stress management, and targeted supplements can go a long way toward helping you achieve better health. But, even if you're doing everything else right, you'll never attain optimal health if you don't change the way you eat. This is because food is truly medicine, and it's more powerful than drugs. And, if you live like most people in Westernized countries, the combination of unhealthy food choices and poor lifestyle habits can set you up for one or more chronic health problems and, quite likely, dying long before you should. In fact, an incredible 98 percent of all disease is caused by a combination of unhealthy food choices and poor lifestyle habits.

· · · · · · · · · ·

Even those in more conventional medical settings are starting to realize that poor nutrition—and not the genes you inherit—is the primary cause of disease and early death in our country. According to Stephen Kopecky, MD, a preventive cardiologist at the Mayo Clinic, having certain genes for a particular disease increases your risk by only 30 to 40 percent, whereas poor food choices and an unhealthy lifestyle can increase your risk by as much as 400 percent!

I truly believe that food can either cure disease or cause disease, based on your choices. From the research I've seen, I'm convinced that you can prevent, improve, and potentially reverse a variety of chronic diseases, including allergies, Alzheimer's and other forms of dementia, anxiety and depression, heart disease, migraines, osteoarthritis, type 2 diabetes, Parkinson's disease, and even some forms of cancer, just by adopting the right dietary choices. That's why I follow a diet that is low in carbohydrates, high in healthy fats, with moderate amounts of high-quality animal protein. If you're sick and tired of being sick and tired, you, too, may reap a wealth of benefits by changing your diet from one that is high in carbohydrates to a diet like mine that is rich in protein and fats.

Look and Feel 20 Years Younger

Earlier in this book, you learned what constitutes a healthy diet—and how the typical Western diet sets the stage for disease.

Now it's time to put that knowledge into practice. Not only will optimizing your diet help prevent you from experiencing a life crippled by disease; it will recharge your health—both inside and out. As a result, you'll look and feel considerably younger than your chronological age.

But this won't happen unless you realize that *your health* is *your responsibility*. No one else can make you healthy. Not your doctor, not your insurance company, and certainly not drug manufacturers. Contrary to the lies that modern medicine spouts, you can't live in a sedentary, fast-food lane and think that prescription and over-the-counter drugs will treat your diseases and make you healthy. Drugs do not promote good health! At best, they merely treat symptoms. In some cases, they can even cause more health problems than they claim to solve. And conventional doctors? They are trained to focus exclusively on disease and never receive an adequate education in the critical roles nutrition and lifestyle play in fostering good health.

But here's the good news: you can absolutely regain your health regardless of your gender, age, or whatever health challenges you face. The key is to embrace healthy choices, starting with the foods you eat day in and day out.

Remember the "garbage in, garbage out" analogy I mentioned in Chapter 2? It turns out that the opposite is also true. When you put high-quality food into your body, you get high-quality results. And this matters because your body completely rebuilds itself at least four times between the time you're born and the time you die.

This includes your heart, liver, bones, and brain (and your brain cells). By providing your body with quality information from the foods you eat, this reconstruction process will yield quality results.

Bottom line—your body is continually renewing your cells. That's why it's critically important to opt for a healthy diet that provides the tools needed to nourish your cells. The result is better health and vitality today, and better odds of a healthy, disease-free tomorrow.

The Keto Connection to Optimal Health

A growing number of human studies are confirming the health benefits of a ketogenic diet. What exactly is a ketogenic diet? At its core, a keto diet is a very low-carb, high-fat, moderate-protein way of eating. It involves replacing much of your carbohydrate consumption with high-quality fats like coconut oil or extra-virgin olive oil, full-fat dairy, and fatty cuts of meat. This triggers a metabolic state called ketosis in which the body becomes incredibly efficient at burning fat for energy. It also turns fat into ketones in the liver. Over time, the body learns to burn these ketones instead of glucose for energy. A ketogenic diet can foster not only rapid weight loss but also significant drops in blood sugar and insulin levels.

The ketogenic diet was originally adopted in the 1920s to treat epilepsy before the advent of anti-seizure medications. While the diet largely fell out of favor because of the convenience these drugs provided, it continued to be used in people who were resistant to anti-seizure medication. But then something interesting happened in 2013. A study published in the journal *Science* reported that the body's powerful antioxidant and anti-inflammatory genes were activated by one particular ketone body called beta-hydroxybutyrate. And this ketone was produced by severely limiting carbohydrate intake. The low-carb keto diet quickly regained popularity because it also induced rapid weight loss. But the real value was its ability to slow the aging process and positively impact a wide range of chronic illnesses.

Keto 1, 2, 3

To reap all the benefits keto has to offer, you can't simply load up on butter and rib eye steaks without making changes to the rest of your diet and lifestyle. Here are the basic principles of a successful ketogenic diet that can help you lose weight, reduce the risk of nearly all chronic conditions, and promote optimal health.

✦ Consume an adequate amount of high-quality (preferably grass-fed, pastured, or wild-caught) animal protein. What's adequate? About 30 percent of your total calories or 1 to 1.5 grams of protein per pound of body weight.

✦ Eat plenty of *natural* fat, ensuring that it makes up 60 to 70 percent of your diet. Excellent sources include animal fats, eggs, olive oil, avocado oil, butter, MCT (medium chain triglyceride) oil, coconut oil, and lard.

✦ Snack on all types of tree nuts, especially almonds and walnuts. Because peanuts are actually a legume, not a nut, they should be avoided.

✦ Highly restrict all carbohydrates to less than 10 percent of your total diet. This translates to approximately 20 to 40 grams daily, not the typical 300 to 400 grams consumed on the Standard American Diet.

✦ Reduce the amount of fruit you eat and absolutely avoid fruit juice as it is typically high in harmful fructose. You can eat low-sugar fruits, such as grapefruit, lemons, limes, and berries in moderation.

✦ Eat low-carb, non-starchy vegetables like greens and most veggies grown above ground. Don't eat roots or tubers, such as beets, carrots, potatoes, or sweet potatoes, as these vegetables are high in starch and carbohydrates.

✦ If desired, enjoy one glass of red wine daily for women and two for men. Studies show that red wine is high in polyphenols, especially resveratrol, anthocyanins, and catechins.

✦ It's absolutely critical to shun all types of sugar—especially high-fructose corn syrup—as well as artificial sweeteners. This means *no* diet soft drinks or low-calorie juices.

✦ Totally avoid *all* grains and refined flours as they are high in carbohydrates, with many being sources of gluten.

✦ Ditch most forms of dairy from cows in favor of dairy from goats.* The exceptions are fermented forms like yogurt and kefir. You may also opt for organic almond or coconut milk as a dairy substitute.

✦ Restrict your daily intake to 2,000 calories or less for women and a maximum of 2,500 calories for men.

✦ To truly maximize the benefits of a keto diet, adopt the following health habits:

✦ Sleep seven to nine hours each night. Consistency is key so strive to go to bed and wake up at the same time every day.

✦ Keep moving. Exercise several times a week for at least 20 to 30 minutes at a time. Choose from walking, swimming, biking, weight training, kettlebell swings, and squats. Or try one of my HIIT routines in Chapter 6.

✦ Manage stress by meditating daily or doing some box breathing as needed.

* Dairy can provide health benefits for some people. However, many are allergic to milk and most people have a difficult time digesting the casein and lactose in cow's milk. Personally, I can't tolerate cow's milk, but I can digest goat's milk—especially unpasteurized (raw) goat's milk. Just be aware that if you consume raw goat's or cow's milk—or any raw animal products—the U.S. Department of Agriculture's Food Safety and Inspection Service notes that "consuming raw or undercooked meats, poultry, seafood, shellfish, or eggs may increase your risk of foodborne illness, especially if you have certain medical conditions."

KETO FOOD CHOICES AT A GLANCE

When choosing the foods for your keto diet, opt for organic whenever possible. Meat and dairy should also ideally come from grass-fed animals. Eggs and poultry should be sourced from pasture-raised organic birds, and fish should be wild-caught, low-mercury varieties.

FOODS YOU SHOULD EAT	FOODS/INGREDIENTS YOU SHOULD AVOID
Beef and lamb	Artificial colors and flavors
Berries and some citrus (lemons, limes, grapefruit)	Artificial sweeteners
Celtic Sea Salt	Beans and legumes
Dairy (full-fat butter, cream, kefir, yogurt)	Beer and sugary mixed drinks
Eggs	Breads and baked goods
Fats and oils (avocado, coconut, olive oil, lard)	Candy and other sweets
Fish and seafood	Fruit (except those noted as acceptable)
Game (bison, elk, rabbit, venison)	Grains and refined flours
Non-starchy vegetables (unlimited amounts)	High-carb sugary sauces and dressings
Pork (including nitrate/nitrite-free bacon)	Pasta, noodles, and rice
Poultry (chicken, duck, turkey, including the skin)	Refined salt
Red wine (in moderation)	Starchy vegetables (potatoes, corn, peas)
Vinegars	Sugar (refined and "natural" varieties)
	Sweetened beverages
	Vegetable and seed oils, margarine

CHAPTER 11

Terry's Sample Meal Plan

To help kick off your new keto diet, I've put together a sample meal plan that adheres to all the guidelines outlined in the previous chapter. Depending on your current way of eating, you might think that these meals are time consuming to prepare. And yes, if you're used to takeout or meals you can just heat up in the microwave, they do take a bit more time. But, when you consider it as an investment in your health, it's time well spent.

• • • • • • • • • •

You'll also notice that the sample meals are heavy on fats and protein while being quite low in carbohydrates. Now, I know that it can be difficult to cut your carbohydrate intake to improve your diet, but it's worth it. Controlling carbs will have the most powerful and meaningful impact on healing and restoring your health. As a bonus, it can also help you lose the weight you always wanted to lose—especially that stubborn belly fat.

Use these tips to help keep your carb intake in check:

✦ Consume no more than 72 grams of carbohydrates daily. For best results, try to reduce your carb intake to 20 to 40 grams per day.

✦ Get your carbohydrates primarily from non-starchy vegetables.

✦ Know the amount of carbohydrates (in grams) in everything you eat and make smart choices. You can find sources online that can give you a reliable carb count for a variety of foods.

A Special Note on Dairy Products

As I've mentioned, I have trouble digesting dairy in most forms. However, if you can tolerate it, I strongly recommend drinking only fresh, raw milk from organically managed cows or goats. Raw dairy products are vastly superior to the pasteurized, hormone-laced products you get at the grocery store. Drinking up to a quart of raw milk daily will supply an exceptional form of high-quality protein, good fats, and numerous enzymes and nutrients that are often destroyed in the heating process.

I also recommend soft-cooked eggs. Eggs are an excellent source of protein and are packed with vitamins, minerals, and carotenoids such as lutein and zeaxanthin.

Don't believe all the bad press eggs have received over the past 40 years. They are wonderful for your health.

YOUR SAMPLE KETO MEAL PLAN

This way of eating works for me—and it can work for you too! And because it's exclusively built around whole, nutrient-dense foods, it gives your body exactly what it needs for vibrant, good health. I've seen it work miracles in my own health and in that of others who have adopted this whole-food, keto way of eating.

BREAKFAST

+ 2–4 eggs, any style and cooked in butter, extra-virgin olive oil, coconut oil, or lard

+ 1/2 grapefruit or other low–glycemic index (GI) fruit

+ 2–4 slices of sugar-free bacon, with no nitrates or nitrites

+ 1 cup of coffee or green tea with whole cream

MIDMORNING SNACK

+ 1/4 cup raw almonds or walnuts
  or
+ 1 hard-boiled egg

LUNCH

+ Meat, poultry, or fish

+ Non-starchy vegetables with lemon juice, Celtic Sea Salt, and olive oil or butter

+ Unsweetened coffee, green tea, or iced tea with lemon

MIDAFTERNOON SNACK

+ 1–2 ounces of goat cheese

+ Small handful of walnuts

DINNER

+ Unlimited salad (lettuce, tomatoes, cucumbers, avocado, bell peppers, mushrooms, etc.) seasoned with olive oil and Celtic Sea Salt

+ Meat, poultry, or fish

+ Steamed broccoli, snow peas, asparagus, or zucchini, dressed with Celtic Sea Salt and either butter or olive oil

DESSERT

+ Berries with full-fat heavy cream

BEDTIME SNACK

+ Small handful of nuts or seeds, and 1 ounce of cheese

PLENTY PRIOR PLANNING = SUCCESS

When you're just starting out, it's smart to plan ahead. Create a menu for at least the next three days (a week may work even better for you) and write out your grocery list. Make sure to include the following keto-friendly foods:

Eggs: Organic or pastured whole eggs are the best choice

Poultry: Chicken, duck, or turkey

Fatty fish: Wild-caught salmon, sardines, herring, or mackerel

Meat: Grass-fed beef, venison, pork, organ meats, bison, or lamb

Full-fat dairy: Yogurt, butter, or cream

Full-fat cheese: Goat cheese, cream cheese, or feta cheese

Nuts and seeds: Macadamia nuts, almonds, walnuts, pumpkin seeds, or flaxseeds

Nut butter: Natural almond or walnut butter

Healthy fats: Extra-virgin olive oil, avocado oil, coconut oil, MCT oil, butter, cream, or lard

Avocados: Whole avocados, which can be added to almost any meal or snack

Non-starchy vegetables: Asparagus, broccoli, Brussels sprouts, cauliflower, green beans, mushrooms, onions, red bell peppers

Condiments: Celtic Sea Salt, pepper, vinegar, lemon juice, fresh herbs and spices

Wine: Particularly red wine—especially malbec, petite sirah, St. Laurent, and pinot noir, which have all been found to contain the highest levels of resveratrol

A WORD ABOUT SNACKING

You may find that, after a few days, you don't really need snacks to help keep you satisfied. That's because, unlike processed carbs, the protein and fat in your meals will keep you satiated for hours. However, even if you take snacks off the table, it's smart to grab a handful of nuts and sneak them into your meals on a daily basis. Nuts, which are loaded with antioxidants and healthy fats, have been shown to reduce inflammation, support cardiovascular health, and improve blood sugar. Plus, they are packed with healthy fiber and protein.

But if you do want to incorporate snacks into your daily meal plan, you have numerous options:

- Almond butter

- Chopped raw vegetables

- Raw goat or feta cheese

- Slices of cold meat, such as turkey, chicken, or roast beef, with mustard or sugar-free salsa

- Half an avocado with raw vegetables

- One or two soft- or hard-boiled eggs

- Tomato slices with fresh sliced mozzarella cheese, drizzled with extra-virgin olive oil and sprinkled with fresh basil

- 2-3 small squares (0.5-1 ounce) of dark chocolate. Just make sure it contains at least 70% cacao.

Resources

CLEAN CONDIMENTS

Chosen Foods. Healthy non-GMO avocado-based cooking sprays, oils, mayonnaise, and salad dressings. *chosenfoods.com*

Primal Kitchen. Avocado-based condiments and sauces that are free from gluten, grains, sugars, and industrially processed oils. *primalkitchen.com*

Red Boat. Fish sauce containing only black anchovies and salt, made using traditional Vietnamese fermentation. *redboatfishsauce.com*

GRASS-FED AND PASTURE-RAISED FOODS

ButcherBox. High-quality grass-fed meat, organic, pasture-raised poultry, and wild-caught seafood. *butcherbox.com*

Grass Roots Farmers' Cooperative. Grass-fed and grass-finished beef and bison, as well as pastured lamb, pork, and poultry. All animals are regeneratively farmed in the United States and raised with no hormones or antibiotics. *grassrootscoop.com*

U.S. Wellness Meats. Owned and run by family farmers, U.S. Wellness Meats offers meat from animals that graze organic grasslands managed through the practice of rotational grazing. *grasslandbeef.com*

HEALTHY STAPLES

Thrive Market. Membership-based store that delivers a wide range of clean and healthy groceries right to your door. For every membership purchased, Thrive Market donates a membership to a low-income family, teacher, student, or veteran. All prices are wholesale. *thrivemarket.com*

Whole Spice. Affordably priced certified-organic kosher herbs and spices, as well as blends. Available for mail order or at their Napa, California store. *wholespice.com*

LOCAL AND ORGANIC PRODUCE

Imperfect Foods. Sustainable and often organic produce and groceries delivered directly to your door. Partners with local farmers to save ugly produce, surplus items, and more from being wasted and ending up in landfills. *imperfectfoods.com*

Local Harvest. A comprehensive database of local farmers and ranchers that offer CSA (community supported agriculture) programs across the U.S. *localharvest.org*

Misfits Market. Works directly with farmers and food producers to source organic produce and high-quality pantry staples, meats, and seafood. Food is delivered to your door weekly in eco-friendly packaging. *misfitsmarket.com*

ORGANIC AND BIODYNAMIC WINE

Dry Farm Wines. Offers a variety of biodynamic, additive-free, sugar-free, low-alcohol wines. This wine club allows you to choose your own varieties and delivers with free shipping. *dryfarmwines.com*

Organic Wine Exchange. Offers a variety of wine clubs, including a biodynamic wine club, an organic wine club, and a sulfite-free wine club. They also have gluten-free wine for those with sensitivities. *organicwineexchange.com*

SAFE AND SUSTAINABLE SEAFOOD

Monterey Bay Aquarium Seafood Watch. Download an easy-to-use guide on which sources of sustainable seafood to choose. *seafoodwatch.org*

PureFish. Offers a wide variety of high-quality, wild-caught, and sustainable seafood, delivered right to your home. *purefish.com*

Sea to Table. Wild-caught, sustainable, traceable seafood originating in U.S. waters and delivered to your doorstep. *sea2table.com*

Vital Choice. Wild-caught fish and seafood from healthy, well-managed fisheries around the globe. Free shipping on all orders. *Vitalchoice.com*

EXERCISE APPS AND EQUIPMENT

DICK'S Sporting Goods. Brick-and-mortar and online shopping. DICK'S carries everything you need to set up a home gym. Their large array of exercise equipment includes free weights and kettlebells, resistance bands, and TRX suspension training systems. *dickssportinggoods.com/c/exercise-equipment*

MIRROR. An interactive mirror that offers over 10,000 on-demand fitness classes, live workouts, and one-on-one training. The MIRROR's sleek, slim design takes up only two feet of wall space, making it an ideal home-gym solution for anyone short on space. Plus, you can access all the workouts on your smartphone for workouts on the go. *shop.lululemon.com/story/mirror-home-gym*

Peloton. Even if you don't purchase one of Peloton's spin bikes or treadmills, you can still tap into its large library of workouts via the Peloton app. For just $12.99 per month, you can access barre, boxing, Pilates, strength training, stretching, and yoga workouts from your laptop, smartphone, or tablet. Plus you can try it for 30 days at no charge. *onepeloton.com*

SLEEP AND STRESS RELIEF

American Massage Therapy Association. A nationwide database of professional massage therapists that can be easily accessed via a simple search. *amtamassage.org/find-massage-therapist*

Apollo Wearables. Developed by neuroscientists and physicians, this wearable stress-relief tool uses therapeutic touch to strengthen and rebalance your autonomic nervous system. The result is better sleep, improved focus, and less stress. *apolloneuro.com*

AromaWeb. Comprehensive site for all things aromatherapy, including a list of online and brick-and-mortar retailers who carry pure essential oils. *aromaweb.com*

Headspace. Mindfulness and meditation app that can effectively help to reduce stress and anxiety. Thousands of meditations and sleep sounds are designed to improve your mental health naturally. *headspace.com*

Komuso Shift. Beautiful breath-work jewelry designed by psychotherapists to help quickly and easily combat anxiety, soothe the feelings of stress, and improve focus by slowing your breathing. *komusodesign.com*

SUPPLEMENTS

Terry Naturally. Research-backed, clinically effective dietary supplements that include botanical blends and proprietary nutritional formulations based on responsibly sourced ingredients from around the world. *europharmausa.com*

ALTERNATIVE MEDICINE PRACTITIONERS AND TESTING

Andrew Weil Center for Integrative Medicine. Integrative medicine looks at the whole patient and uses evidence-based therapies from both the world of conventional and the world of alternative medicines. This center maintains a comprehensive database of integrative medicine doctors throughout the U.S. and Canada. *integrativemedicine.arizona.edu/alumni.html*

The Institute for Functional Medicine. Functional medicine doctors look beyond symptoms to uncover the root cause of disease. They typically use nutrition and alternative practices to heal the underlying issue instead of simply treating symptoms. IFM maintains a searchable database to help you find a functional medicine doctor in your area. *ifm.org/find-a-practitioner*

Cell Science Systems. This lab offers several tests that can be ordered by either a physician or a patient. These include the ALCAT food-sensitivity test, a telomere length test, and a cellular nutritional assay. *cellsciencesystems.com*

Oxford Biomedical Technologies. Offering the LEAP MRT food-sensitivity test that measures the inflammatory response to various foods. This lab provides a complimentary prescreening to see if MRT testing might be right for you. *nowleap.com/the-patented-mediator-release-test*

ORGANIZATIONS AND MEDIA

Environmental Working Group. Research and environmental advocacy group with consumer guides on food, personal care, and water safety, including the Dirty Dozen and Clean Fifteen produce guides. *ewg.org*

Ketogenic Diet Resource. This site provides a wealth of information on the mechanics of the ketogenic diet and how it can benefit health. *ketogenic-diet-resource.com*

Organic Consumers Association. Information regarding organic initiatives and legislation, as well as product information. *organicconsumer.org*

Terry Talks Nutrition. Articles, blog posts, podcasts, and videos spanning a comprehensive range of health topics. If you want more of my perspectives on health, this is the place. *terrytalksnutrition.com*

RECOMMENDED READING

Breaking the Vicious Cycle: Intestinal Health through Diet by Elaine Gottschall, BA, MS

Eat Fat, Lose Fat: Lose Weight and Feel Great with the Delicious, Science-Based Coconut Diet by Mary Enig, PhD, and Sally Fallon

Grain Brain: The Surprising Truth about Wheat, Carbs, and Sugar—Your Brain's Silent Killers by David Perlmutter, MD

Iodine: Why You Need It, Why You Can't Live without It by David Brownstein, MD

Know Your Fats: The Complete Primer for Understanding the Nutrition of Fats, Oils, and Cholesterol by Mary Enig, PhD

Life Without Bread: How a Low-Carbohydrate Diet Can Save Your Life by Christian B. Allan, PhD, and Wolfgang Lutz, MD

Lipitor, Thief of Memory: Statin Drugs and the Misguided War on Cholesterol by Duane Graveline, MD

Overcoming Thyroid Disorders by David Brownstein, MD

Statin Drugs Side Effects and the Misguided War on Cholesterol by Duane Graveline, MD

The Great Cholesterol Con: The Truth about What Really Causes Heart Disease and How to Avoid It by Malcolm Kendrick, GP

The Paleo Diet: Lose Weight and Get Healthy by Eating the Foods You Were Designed to Eat by Loren Cordain, PhD

Vitamin B6 Therapy: Nature's Versatile Healer by John M. Ellis, MD, and Jean Pamplin

Wheat Belly: Lose the Wheat, Lose the Weight, and Find Your Path Back to Health by William Davis, MD

References

■ **PREFACE**

Buttorff C, Ruder T, Bauman M. "Multiple Chronic Conditions in the United States." RAND Corporation. 2017. https://www.rand.org/pubs/tools/TL221.html.

Centers for Disease Control and Prevention. 2021. www.cdc.gov/chronicdisease/index.htm

Raghupathi W, Raghupathi V. An empirical study of chronic diseases in the United States: a visual analytics approach to public health. *International Journal of Environmental Research and Public Health*. 2018;15(3):431.

■ **INTRODUCTION**

Alegria-Torres JA, Baccarelli A, Bollarti V. Epigenetics and lifestyle. *Epigenomics*. 2011;3(3):267–77.

Ali A, Katz DL. Disease prevention and health promotion: how integrative medicine fits. *American Journal of Preventive Medicine*. 2015;49(5 Supp 3):S230–40.

Barreto FM. Beneficial effects of *Lactobacillus plantarum* on glycemia and homocysteine levels in postmenopausal women with metabolic syndrome. *Nutrition*. 2014;30(7–8):939–42.

Chakraborty SP. Patho-physiological and toxicological aspects of monosodium glutamate. *Toxicology Mechanisms and Methods*. 2019;29(6):389–96.

Das T, Jayasudha R, Chakravarthy S, et al. Alterations in the gut bacterial microbiome in people with type 2 diabetes mellitus and diabetic retinopathy. *Scientific Reports*. 2021;11:2738.

Dedoussis G, Kaliora AC, Panagiotakos DB. Genes, diet and type 2 diabetes mellitus: a review. *The Review of Diabetic Studies*. 2007;4(1):13–24.

Felsenfeld G. A brief history of epigenetics. *Cold Spring Harbor Perspectives in Biology*. 2014;6(1):a018200.

Ferguson JF, Allayee H, Gerszten RE, et al. Nutrigenomics, the microbiome, and gene-environment interactions: new directions in cardiovascular disease research, prevention, and treatment. *Circulation Cardiovascular Genetics*. 2016;9:291–313.

Haro D, Marrero PF, Relat J. Nutritional regulation of gene expression: carbohydrate-, fat-, and amino acid–dependent modulation of transcriptional activity. *International Journal of Molecular Sciences*. 2019;20(6):1386.

Hellman BA. Gut bacteria gene complement dwarfs human genome. *Nature*. 2010;464:7285.

Kvaavik E, Batty GD, Ursin G, et al. Influence of individual and combined health behaviors on total and cause-specific mortality in men and women: the United Kingdom health and lifestyle survey. *Archives of Internal Medicine*. 2010;170(8):711–8.

Langkamp-Henken B, Rowe CC, Ford AL, et al. *Bifidobacterium bifidum* R0071 results in a greater proportion of healthy days and a lower percentage of academically stressed students reporting a day of cold/flu: a randomised, double-blind, placebo-controlled study. *British Journal of Nutrition*. 2015;113(3):426–34.

Li Y, Pan A, Wang DD, et al. Impact of healthy lifestyle factors on life expectancies in the US population. *Circulation*. 2018;138(4):345–55.

Luck H, Khan S, Kim JH, et al. Gut-associated IgA immune cells regulate obesity-related insulin resistance. *Nature Communications*. 2019;10(1).

Marcon F, Siniscalchi E, Crebelli R, et al. Diet-related telomere shortening and chromosome stability. *Mutagenesis*. 2012;27(1):49–57.

Marizzoni M, Cattaneo A, Mirabelli P, et al. Short-chain fatty acids and lipopolysaccharide as mediators between gut dysbiosis and amyloid pathology in Alzheimer's disease. *Journal of Alzheimer's Disease*. 2020;78(2):683.

Ouwehand AC, Bergsma N, Parhiala R. *Bifidobacterium* microbiota and parameters of immune function in elderly subjects. *FEMS Immunology & Medical Microbiology*. 2008;53(1):18–25.

Rodriguez-Palacios A, Harding A, Menghini P, et al. The artificial sweetener Splenda promotes gut proteobacteria, dysbiosis, and myeloperoxidase reactivity in Crohn's disease-like ileitis. *Inflammatory Bowel Disease*. 2018;24(5):1005–20.

Saccharin: Review of safety issues. *JAMA*. 1985;254 (18):2622–4.

Scheithauer T, Rampanelli E, Nieuwdorp M, et al. Gut microbiota as a trigger for metabolic inflammation in obesity and type 2 diabetes. *Frontiers in Immunology*. 2020;11:571731.

Sharma P, Bhardwaj P, Singh R. Administration of *Lactobacillus casei* and *Bifidobacterium bifidum* ameliorated hyperglycemia, dyslipidemia, and oxidative stress in diabetic rats. *International Journal of Preventive Medicine*. 2016;7:102.

Sharma S, Tripathi P. Gut microbiome and type 2 diabetes: where we are and where to go? *Journal of Nutritional Biochemistry*. 2019;63:101–8.

Sonestedt E, Hellstrand S, Schulz CA, et al. The association between carbohydrate-rich foods and risk of cardiovascular disease is not modified by genetic susceptibility to dyslipidemia as determined by 80 validated variants. *PLOS ONE*. 2015;10(4):e0126104.

Trøseid M, Andersen GØ, Broch, K, et al. The gut microbiome in coronary artery disease and heart failure: current knowledge and future directions. *EBioMedicine*. 2020;52:102649.

"Ultra-processed food consumption is associated with chromosomal changes linked to biological ageing." EurekAlert! 2020. https://www.eurekalert.org/news-releases/ 487842.

Valdes AM, Walter J, Segal E, et al. Role of the gut microbiota in nutrition and health. *BMJ*. 2018;361:k2179.

Voruganti VS. Nutritional genomics of cardiovascular disease. *Current Genetic Medicine Reports*. 2018;6(2):98–106.

Wang B, Xu H, Wei H, et al. Oral administration of *Bifidobacterium bifidum* for modulating microflora, acid and bile resistance, and physiological indices in mice. *Canadian Journal of Microbiology*. 2015;61(2):155–63.

Xu H, Wang J, Cai J, et al. Protective effect of *Lactobacilus rhamnosus* GG and its supernatant against myocardial dysfunction in obese mice exposed to intermittent hypoxia is associated with the activation of Nrf2 pathway. *International Journal of Biological Sciences*. 2019;15(11):2471–83.

■ CHAPTER 1

Barth CR, Funchal GA, Luft C, et al. Carrageenan-induced inflammation promotes ROS generation and neutrophil extracellular trap formation in a mouse model of peritonitis. *European Journal of Immunology*. 2016 Apr;46(4):964–70.

Cawley J, Meyerhoefer C. The medical care costs of obesity: an instrumental variables approach. *Journal of Health Economics*. 2012;31(1):219–30.

Chen X, Zhang Z, Yang H, et al. Consumption of ultra-processed foods and health outcomes: a systematic review of epidemiological studies. *Nutrition Journal*. 2020;19:86.

Chiuve SE, Willett WC. The 2005 Food Guide Pyramid: an opportunity lost? *Nature Clinical Practice: Cardiovascular Medicine*. 2007;4(11):610–20.

Comparsi B, Meinerz DF, Franco JL, et al. Diphenyl ditelluride targets brain selenoproteins in vivo: inhibition of cerebral thioredoxin reductase and glutathione peroxidase in mice after acute exposure. *Molecular and Cellular Biochemistry*. 2012;370(1–2):173–82.

Dor A, Ferguson C, Langwith C, et al. "A heavy burden: The individual costs of being overweight and obese in the United States." The George Washington University Department of Health Policy Research. 2010. https://www.researchgate.net/publication/266499190_A_Heavy_Burden_The_Individual_Costs_of_Being_Overweight_and_Obese_in_the_United_States.

Gearhardt AN, Hebebrand J. The concept of "food addiction" helps inform the understanding of overeating and obesity: YES. *American Journal of Clinical Nutrition*. 2021;113(2):263–7.

"GMO Crops, Animal Food, and Beyond." U.S. Food & Drug Administration. 2020. https://www.fda.gov/

food/agricultural-biotechnology/gmo-crops-animal-food-and-beyond.

Hall KD, Ayuketah A, Brychta R, et al. Ultra-processed diets cause excess calorie intake and weight gain: an inpatient randomized controlled trial of ad libitum food intake. *Cell Metabolism*. 2019;30(1):67–77.e3.

Hebebrand J, Gearhardt AN. The concept of "food addiction" helps inform the understanding of overeating and obesity: NO. *American Journal of Clinical Nutrition*. 2021;113(2):268–73.

Kapczuk P, Komorniak N, Rogulska K, et al. Highly processed food and its effect on health of children and adults. *Postepy Biochem*. 2020;66(1):23–9.

Katz DL, Meller S. Can we say what diet is best for health? *Annual Review of Public Health*. 2014;35:83–103.

Kearns K, Dee A, Fitzgerald AP, et al. Chronic disease burden associated with overweight and obesity in Ireland: the effects of a small BMI reduction at population level. *BMC Public Health*. 2014;14:143.

Lustig RH. Ultraprocessed food: addictive, toxic, and ready for regulation. *Nutrients*. 2020;12(11):3401.

Nestle M. Food lobbies, the food pyramid, and U.S. nutrition policy. *International Journal of Health Services*. 1993;23(3):483–96.

Nyberg ST, Batty GD, Pentti J, et al. Obesity and loss of disease-free years owing to major non-communicable diseases: a multicohort study. *Lancet Public Health*. 2018;3(10):e490–7.

Pi-Sunyer X. The medical risks of obesity. *Postgraduate Medicine*. 2009;121(6):21–33.

Schulte EM, Avena NM, Gearhardt AN. Which foods may be addictive? The roles of processing, fat content, and glycemic load. *PLOS ONE*. 2015;10(2):e0117959.

Vojdani A, Vojdani C. Immune reactivity to food coloring. *Alternative Therapies in Health and Medicine*. 2015;21(Suppl 1):52–62.

CHAPTER 2

Andersson A, Tengblad S, Karlström B, et al. Whole-grain foods do not affect insulin sensitivity or markers of lipid peroxidation and inflammation in healthy, moderately overweight subjects. *The Journal of Nutrition*. 2007;137(6):1401–7.

Arnold LE, Lofthouse N, Hurt E. Artificial food colors and attention-deficit/hyperactivity symptoms: conclusions to dye for. *Neurotherapeutics*. 2012;9(3):599–609.

Bahadoran Z, Ghasemi A, Mirmiran P, et al. Nitrate-nitrite-nitrosamines exposure and the risk of type 1 diabetes: a review of current data. *World Journal of Diabetes*. 2016;7(18):433–40.

Bhatnagar S, Aggarwal R. Lactose intolerance. *BMJ*. 2007;334(7608):1331–2.

Bian X, Chi L, Gao B, et al. The artificial sweetener acesulfame potassium affects the gut microbiome and body weight gain in CD-1 mice. *PLOS ONE*. 2017;12(6):e0178426.

Boyd ES, Pike MC, Short RV, et al. Women's reproductive cancers in evolutionary context. *The Quarterly Review of Biology*. 1994;69(3):353–67.

Davidson TL, Chan K, Jarrard LE, et al. Contributions of the hippocampus and medial prefrontal cortex to energy and body weight regulation. *Hippocampus*. 2009;19(3):235–52.

de Punder K, Pruimboom L. The dietary intake of wheat and other cereal grains and their role in inflammation. *Nutrients*. 2013;5(3):771–87.

DiNicolantonio JJ, O'Keefe JH. Importance of maintaining a low omega-6/omega-3 ratio for reducing inflammation. *Open Heart*. 2018;5(2):e000946.

Feferman L, Bhattacharyya S, Oates E, et al. Carrageenan-free diet shows improved glucose tolerance and insulin signaling in prediabetes: a randomized, pilot clinical trial. *Journal of Diabetes Research*. 2020;2020:8267980.

Feskanich D, Willett WC, Stampfer MJ, et al. Milk, dietary calcium, and bone fractures in women: a 12-year prospective study. *American Journal of Public Health*. 1997;87(6):992–7.

Freed DL. Do dietary lectins cause disease?. *BMJ*. 1999;318(7190):1023–4.

Gurven MD, Trumble BC, Stieglitz J, et al. Cardiovascular disease and type 2 diabetes in evolutionary perspective: a critical role for helminths? *Evolution, Medicine, and Public Health*. 2016;2016(1):338–57.

Han SN, Leka LS, Lichtenstein AH, et al. Effect of hydrogenated and saturated, relative to polyunsaturated, fat on immune and inflammatory responses of adults with moderate hypercholesterolemia. *Journal of Lipid Research*. 2002;43(3):445–52.

Hollon J, Puppa EL, Greenwald B, et al. Effect of gliadin on permeability of intestinal biopsy explants from celiac disease patients and patients with non-celiac gluten sensitivity. *Nutrients*. 2015;7(3):1565–76.

Hori Y, Ihara N, Teramoto N, et al. Noninvasive quantification of cerebral metabolic rate for glucose in rats using ^{18}F-FDG PET and standard input function. *Journal of Cerebral Blood Flow & Metabolism*. 2015;35(10):1664–70.

Hu FB, Manson JE, Stampfer MJ, et al. Diet, lifestyle, and the risk of type 2 diabetes mellitus in women. *New England Journal of Medicine*. 2001;345(11):790–7.

Jacobs ET, Foote JA, Kohler LN, et al. Re-examination of dairy as a single commodity in US dietary guidance. *Nutrition Reviews*. 2020;78(3):225–34.

Jakszyn P, Gonzalez CA. Nitrosamine and related food intake and gastric and oesophageal cancer risk: a systematic review of the epidemiological evidence. *World Journal of Gastroenterology*. 2006;12(27):4296–303.

Junker Y, Zeissig S, Kim S, et al. Wheat amylase trypsin inhibitors drive intestinal inflammation via activation of toll-like receptor 4. *Journal of Experimental Medicine*. 2012;209(13):239502408.

Karakula-Juchnowicz H, Rog J, Juchnowicz D, et al. The study evaluating the effect of probiotic supplementation on the mental status, inflammation, and intestinal barrier in major depressive disorder patients using gluten-free or gluten-containing diet (SANGUT study): a 12-week, randomized, double-blind, and placebo-controlled clinical study protocol. *Nutrition Journal*. 2019;18(1):50.

Lopez HW, Leenhardt F, Coudry C, et al. Minerals and phytic acid interactions: is it a real problem for human nutrition? *International Journal of Food Science & Technology*. 2002;37(7):727–39.

Mumolo MG, Rettura F, Melissari S, et al. Is gluten the only culprit for non-celiac gluten/wheat sensitivity? *Nutrients*. 2020;12(12):3785.

Mozaffarian D, Aro A, Willett WC. Health effects of trans-fatty acids: experimental and observational evidence. *European Journal of Clinical Nutrition*. 2009;63(Suppl 2):S5–21.

Nettleton JE, Reimer RA, Shearer J. Reshaping the gut microbiota: impact of low calorie sweeteners and the link to insulin resistance? *Physiology & Behavior*. 2016;164(Pt B):488–93.

O'Keefe S, Gaskins-Wright S, Wiley V, et al. Levels of *trans* geometrical isomers of essential fatty acids in some unhydrogenated U.S. vegetable oils. *Journal of Food Lipids*. 1994;1(3):165–76.

Palmnäs MS, Cowan TE, Bomhof MR, et al. Low-dose aspartame consumption differentially affects gut microbiota-host metabolic interactions in the diet-induced obese rat. *PLOS ONE*. 2014;9(10):e109841.

Pang MD, Goossens GH, Blaak EE. The impact of artificial sweeteners on body weight control and glucose homeostasis. *Frontiers in Nutrition*. 2020;7:598340.

Pearlman M, Obert J, Casey L. The association between artificial sweeteners and obesity. *Current Gastroenterology Reports*. 2017;19:64

Pontzer H, Wood BM, Raichlen DA. Hunter-gatherers as models in public health. *Obesity Reviews*. 2018;19(Suppl 1):24–35.

"Recombinant Bovine Growth Hormone." American Cancer Society. 2014. https://www.cancer.org/cancer/cancer-causes/recombinant-bovine-growth-hormone.html.

Rippe JM, Angelopoulos TJ. Relationship between added sugars consumption and chronic disease risk factors: Current understanding. *Nutrients*. 2016;8(11):697.

Sales IMS, Silva JM, Moura ESR, et al. Toxicity of synthetic flavorings, nature identical and artificial, to hematopoietic tissue cells of rodents. *Brazilian Journal of Biology*. 2018;78(2):306–10.

Salviano Dos Santos VP, Medeiros Salgado A, Guedes Torres A, et al. Benzene as a chemical hazard in processed foods. *International Journal of Food Science*. 2015;2015:545640.

Shanmugalingam T, Bosco C, Ridley AJ, et al. Is there a role for IGF-1 in the development of second primary cancers? *Cancer Medicine*. 2016;5(11):3353–67.

Simon BR, Parlee SD, Learman BS, et al. Artificial sweeteners stimulate adipogenesis and suppress lipolysis independently of sweet taste receptors. *J Biol Chem*. 2013;288(45):32475–89.

Simopoulos AP. An increase in the omega-6/omega-3 fatty acid ratio increases the risk for obesity. *Nutrients*. 2016;8(3):128.

Simopoulos AP. The importance of the ratio of omega-6/omega-3 essential fatty acids. *Biomedical Pharmacotherapy*. 2002;56(8):365–79.

Stanhope KL, Schwarz JM, Keim NL, et al. Consuming fructose-sweetened, not glucose-sweetened, beverages increases visceral adiposity and lipids and decreases insulin sensitivity in overweight/obese humans. *Journal of Clinical Investigation*. 2009;119(5):1322–34.

Stevens LJ, Kuczek T, Burgess JR, et al. Dietary sensitivities and ADHD symptoms: thirty-five years of research. *Clinical Pediatrics (Phila)*. 2011;50(4):279–93.

Suez J, Korem T, Zeevi D, et al. Artificial sweeteners induce glucose intolerance by altering the gut microbiota. *Nature*. 2014;514(7521):181–6.

Sun Q, Ma J, Campos H, et al. A prospective study of trans fatty acids in erythrocytes and risk of coronary heart disease. *Circulation*. 2007;115(14):1858–65.

Vogel KA, Martin BR, McCabe LD, et al. The effect of dairy intake on bone mass and body composition in early pubertal girls and boys: a randomized controlled trial. *American Journal of Clinical Nutrition*. 2017;105(5):1214–29.

Vojdani A. Lectins, agglutinins, and their roles in autoimmune reactivities. *Alternative Therapies in Health and Medicine*. 2015;21(Suppl 1):46–51.

Willet WC, Ludwig DS. Milk and health. *The New England Journal of Medicine*. 2020;382:644–54.

Winterdahl, M, Noer O, Orlowski D, et al. Sucrose intake lowers μ-opioid and dopamine D2/3 receptor availability in porcine brain. *Scientific Reports*. 2019;9:16918.

Yang Q, Zhang Z, Gregg EW, et al. Added sugar intake and cardiovascular diseases mortality among US adults. *JAMA Internal Medicine*. 2014;174(4):516–24.

Zhu Y, Bo Y, Liu Y. Dietary total fat, fatty acids intake, and risk of cardiovascular disease: a dose-response meta-analysis of cohort studies. *Lipids in Health and Disease*. 2019;18(1):91.

Zimmermann MB, Hurrell RF. Nutritional iron deficiency. *Lancet*. 2007;370(9586):511–20.

■ CHAPTER 3

Chapman CL. High-fructose corn syrup-sweetened soft drink consumption increases vascular resistance in the kidneys at rest and during sympathetic activation. *American Journal of Physiology: Renal Physiology*. 2020;318(4):F1053–65.

Danby FW. Nutrition and aging skin: sugar and glycation. *Clinical Dermatology*. 2010;28(4):409–11.

DeChristopher LR. Intake of high-fructose corn syrup sweetened soft drinks, fruit drinks and apple juice is associated with prevalent arthritis in US adults, aged 20–30 years. *Nutrition and Diabetes*. 2016;6(3):e199.

de Souza RJ, Mente A, Maroleanu A, et al. Intake of saturated and trans unsaturated fatty acids and risk of all-cause mortality, cardiovascular disease, and type 2 diabetes: systematic review and meta-analysis of observational studies. *BMJ*. 2015;351:h3978.

Freemas JA. Arterial stiffness is not acutely modified by consumption of a caffeinated soft drink sweetened with high-fructose corn syrup in young healthy adults. *Physiology Reports*. 2021;9(7):e14777.

Ginter E, Simko V. New data on harmful effects of trans-fatty acids. *Bratisl Lek Listy*. 2016;117(5):251–3.

Miao H. Sugar in beverages and the risk of incident dementia, Alzheimer's disease, and stroke: a prospective cohort study. *The Journal of Prevention of Alzheimer's Disease*. 2021;2(8):188–93.

Nestle M. Food lobbies, the food pyramid, and U.S. nutrition policy. *International Journal of Health Services*. 1993;23(3):483–96.

Oteng AB, Kersten S. Mechanisms of action of trans fatty acids. *Advances in Nutrition*. 2020;11(3):697–708.

Price CA. Plasma fatty acid ethanolamides are associated with postprandial triglycerides, ApoCIII, and ApoE in humans consuming a high-fructose corn syrup-sweetened beverage. *American Journal of Physiology, Endocrinology, and Metabolism*. 2018;315(2):E141–9.

Rippe JM, Angelopoulos TJ. Relationship between added sugars consumption and chronic disease risk factors: current understanding. *Nutrients*. 2016;8(11):697.

Siri-Tarino PW, Sun Q, Hu FB, et al. Meta-analysis of prospective cohort studies evaluating the association of saturated fat with cardiovascular disease. *American Journal of Clinical Nutrition*. 2010;91(3):535–46.

Spagnuolo MS. Sweet but bitter: focus on fructose impact on brain function in rodent models. *Nutrients*. 2020;13(1):1.

Stanhope KL. A dose-response study of consuming high-fructose corn syrup-sweetened beverages on lipid/lipoprotein risk factors for cardiovascular disease in young adults. *American Journal of Clinical Nutrition.* 2015;101(6):1144–54.

Wang Y. Phosphorylation and Recruitment of BAF60c in chromatin remodeling for lipogenesis in response to insulin. *Molecular Cell.* 2012;49(2):283–97.

"WHO plan to eliminate industrially-produced trans-fatty acids from global food supply." World Health Organization. 2018. https://www.who.int/news/item/14-05-2018-who-plan-to-eliminate-industrially-produced-trans-fatty-acids-from-global-food-supply.

■ CHAPTER 4

Acker WW, Plasek JM, Blumenthal KG, et al. Prevalence of food allergies and intolerances documented in electronic health records. *Journal of Allergy and Clinical Immunology.* 2017;140(6):1587–91.

Al-Rabia MW. Food-induced immunoglobulin E-mediated allergic rhinitis. *Journal of Microscopy and Ultrastructure.* 2016;4(2):69–75.

Bindslev-Jensen C. Food allergy. *BMJ.* 1998;316(7140): 1299–1302.

Crowe SE. Food allergy vs food intolerance in patients with irritable bowel syndrome. *Gastroenterology & Hepatology.* 2019;15(1):38–40.

Caminero A, Meisel M, Jabri B, et al. Mechanisms by which gut microorganisms influence food sensitivities. *Nature Reviews: Gastroenterology & Hepatology.* 2019;16(1):7-18.

Di Stefano M, Pesatori EV, Manfredi GF, et al. Non-celiac gluten sensitivity in patients with severe abdominal pain and bloating: the accuracy of ALCAT 5. *Clinical Nutrition ESPEN.* 2019;28:127–31.

"Food intolerance." National Health Services. 2019. https://www.nhs.uk/conditions/food-intolerance.

Garcia-Martinez I, Weiss TR, Yousaf MN, et al. A leukocyte activation test identifies food items which induce release of DNA by innate immune peripheral blood leucocytes. *Nutrition & Metabolism.* 2018;15:26.

Gargano D, Appanna R, Santonicola A, et al. Food allergy and intolerance: a narrative review on nutritional concerns. *Nutrients.* 2021;13(5):1638.

Humbert P, Pelletier F, Dreno B, et al. Gluten intolerance and skin diseases. *European Journal of Dermatology.* 2006;16(1):4–11.

Kaczmarki M, Pasula M, Sawicka E, et al. MRT-test—a new generation of tests for food hypersensitivity in children and adults. *Przeglad Pediactryczny.* 1997;1:61–5.

Kelso JM. Unproven diagnostic tests for adverse reactions to foods. *Journal of Allergy and Clinical Immunology: In Practice.* 2017;6(2):362.

König B, Koch AN, Bellanti JA. Studies of mitochondrial and nuclear DNA released from food allergen-activated neutrophils. Implications for non-IgE food allergy. *Allergy and Asthma Proceedings.* 2021;42(3):e59–70.

Lavine E. Blood testing for sensitivity, allergy or intolerance to food. *CMAJ.* 2012;184(6):666–8.

Mullin GE, Swift KM, Lipski L, et al. Testing for food reactions: the good, the bad, and the ugly. *Nutrition in Clinical Practice.* 2010;25(2):192–8.

Nascimento G, Locatelli J, Freitas PC, et al. Antibacterial activity of plant extracts and phytochemicals on antibiotic-resistant bacteria. *Brazilian Journal of Microbiology.* 2000;31:247–56.

Pompei P, Grappasonni I, Scuri S, et al. A clinical evidence of a correlation between insulin resistance and the ALCAT Food Intolerance Test. *Alternative Therapies in Health and Medicine.* 2019;25(2):22–38.

Rotondi AV, Fasano A, Mazzarella G. Non-celiac gluten sensitivity: How its gut immune activation and potential dietary management differ from celiac disease. *Molecular Nutrition & Food Research.* 2018;62(9):e1700854.

Selma MV, Espin, JC, Tomás-Barberán FA. Interaction between phenolics and gut microbiota: role in human health. *Journal of Agricultural and Food Chemistry.* 2009;57(15):6485–501.

Shakoor Z, AlFaifi A, AlAmro B, et al. Prevalence of IgG-mediated food intolerance among patients with allergic symptoms. *Annals of Saudi Medicine.* 2016;36(6):386–90.

"The Food Allergy Epidemic: Facts and Statistics." Food Allergy Research & Education (FARE). 2020. https://www.foodallergy.org/resources/facts-and-statistics.

Wantke F, Götz M, Jarisch R. Histamine-free diet: treatment of choice for histamine-induced food intolerance and supporting treatment for chronic headaches. *Clinical and Experimental Allergy.* 1993;23(12):982–5.

Xie Y, Zhou G, Xu Y, et al. Effects of diet based on IgG elimination combined with probiotics on migraine plus irritable bowel syndrome. *Pain Research & Management*. 2019;2019:7890461.

■ CHAPTER 5

Allen AR, Gullixson LR, Wolhart SC, et al. Dietary sodium influences the effect of mental stress on heart rate variability: a randomized trial in healthy adults. *Journal of Hypertension*. 2014;32(2):374–82.

Andrade AC, Cesena FH, Consolim-Colombo FM, et al. Short-term red wine consumption promotes differential effects on plasma levels of high-density lipoprotein cholesterol, sympathetic activity, and endothelial function in hypercholesterolemic, hypertensive, and healthy subjects. *Clinics (Sao Paulo)*. 2009;64(5):435–42.

Ayee M, Levitan I. Dyslipidemia induced endothelial stiffening is accompanied by increased membrane tension. *Biophysical Journal*. 2019;116:165a.

Battaglia RE, Baumer B, Conrad B, et al. Health risks associated with meat consumption: a review of epidemiological studies. *International Journal for Vitamin and Nutrition Research*. 2015;85(1–2):70–8.

Berrazaga I, Micard V, Gueugneau M, et al. The role of the anabolic properties of plant- versus animal-based protein sources in supporting muscle mass maintenance: a critical review. *Nutrients*. 2019; 11(8):1825.

Białek A, Tokarz A. Conjugated linoleic acid as a potential protective factor in prevention of breast cancer. *Postepy Hig Med Dosw (Online)*. 2013;67:6–14.

Bina J. Dr Lewis Kitchener Dahl, the Dahl rats, and the "inconvenient truth" about the genetics of hypertension. *Hypertension*. 2015;65:963–9.

Bjorntorp P. Importance of fat as a support nutrient for energy: metabolism of athletes. *Journal of Sports Science*. 1991;9(Supp 1):71–6.

Blankson H, Stakkestad JA, Fagertun H, et al. Conjugated linoleic acid reduces body fat mass in overweight and obese humans. *Journal of Nutrition*. 2000;130(12):2943–8.

Burton-Freeman BM, Sandhu AK, Edirisinghe I. Red raspberries and their bioactive polyphenols: cardiometabolic and neuronal health links. *Advances in Nutrition*. 2016;7(1):44–65.

Castro-Webb N, Ruiz-Narváez EA, Campos H. Cross-sectional study of conjugated linoleic acid in adipose tissue and risk of diabetes. *American Journal of Clinical Nutrition*. 2012;96(1):175–81.

Chowdhury R, Warnakula S, Kunutsor S, et al. Association of dietary, circulating, and supplement fatty acids with coronary risk: a systematic review and meta-analysis. *Annals of Internal Medicine*. 2014;160(6):398–406.

Crinnion WJ. Organic food contains higher levels of certain nutrients, lower levels of pesticides, and may provide health benefits to the consumer. *Alternative Medicine Review*. 2010;15(1):4–12.

Daley CA, Abbott A, Doyle, PS, et al. A review of fatty acid profiles and antioxidant content in grass-fed and grain-fed beef. *Nutrition Journal*. 2010;9:10.

Descalzo AM, Rossetti L, Grigioni G, et al. Antioxidant status and odour profile in fresh beef from pasture or grain-fed cattle. *Meat Science*. 2007;75(2):299–307.

Devore EE, Kang JH, Breteler, M, et al. Dietary intakes of berries and flavonoids in relation to cognitive decline. *Annals of Neurology*. 2012;72(1):135–43.

Di Noia J. Defining powerhouse fruits and vegetables: a nutrient density approach. *Preventing Chronic Disease*. 2014;11:130390.

Dreher ML, Davenport AJ. Hass avocado composition and potential health effects. *Critical Reviews in Food Science and Nutrition*. 2013;53(7):738–50.

Duedahl-Olesen L, Ionas AC. Formation and mitigation of PAHs in barbecued meat - a review. *Critical Reviews in Food Science & Nutrition*. 2021;7:1–16.

Estruch R, Ros E, Salas-Salvadó J, et al. Primary prevention of cardiovascular disease with a Mediterranean diet supplemented with extra-virgin olive oil or nuts. *The New England Journal of Medicine*. 2018;378:e34.

Flores M, Saravia C, Vergara CE, et al. Avocado oil: characteristics, properties, and applications. *Molecules*. 2019;24(11):2172.

Garg R, Williams GH, Hurwitz S, et al. Low-salt diet increases insulin resistance in healthy subjects. *Metabolism*. 2011;60(7):965–8.

Gatellier P, Mercier Y, Renerre M. Effect of diet finishing mode (pasture or mixed diet) on antioxidant status of Charolais bovine meat. *Meat Science*. 2004;67(3):385–94.

Gea A, Beunza JJ, Estruch R, et al. Alcohol intake, wine consumption and the development of depression: the PREDIMED study. *BMC Medicine*. 2013;11:192.

Giacosa A, Barale R, Bavaresco L, et al. Mediterranean way of drinking and longevity. *Critical Reviews of Food Science and Nutrition*. 2016;56(4):635–40.

González OA, Escamilla C, Danaher RJ, et al. Antibacterial effects of blackberry extract target periodontopathogens. *Journal of Periodontal Research*. 2013;48(1):80–6.

Graudal N. A radical sodium reduction policy is not supported by randomized controlled trials or observational studies: grading the evidence. *American Journal of Hypertension*. 2016;29(5):543–8.

Honikel KO. The use and control of nitrate and nitrite for the processing of meat products. *Meat Science*. 2008;78(1–2):68–76.

Huang Z, Wang B, Eaves DH, et al. Phenolic compound profile of selected vegetables frequently consumed by African Americans in the southeast United States. *Food Chemistry*. 2007;103(4):1395–402.

Hudthagosol C, Haddad EH, McCarthy K, et al. Pecans acutely increase plasma postprandial antioxidant capacity and catechins and decrease LDL oxidation in humans. *Journal of Nutrition*. 2011;141(1):56–62.

Jafarirad S, Ayoobi N, Karandish M, et al. Dark chocolate effect on serum adiponectin, biochemical and inflammatory parameters in diabetic patients: a randomized clinical trial. *International Journal of Preventive Medicine*. 2018;9:86.

John EM, Stern MC, Sinha R, et al. Meat consumption, cooking practices, meat mutagens, and risk of prostate cancer. *Nutrition and Cancer*. 2011;63(4):525–37.

Khan N, Syed DN, Ahmad N, et al. Fisetin: a dietary antioxidant for health promotion. *Antioxidant & Redox Signaling*. 2013;19(2):151–62.

Kim SR, Kim K, Lee SA, et al. Effect of red, processed, and white meat consumption on the risk of gastric cancer: an overall and dose-response meta-analysis. *Nutrients*. 2019;11(4):826.

Krikorian R, Shidler MD, Nash TA, et al. Blueberry supplementation improves memory in older adults. *Journal of Agricultural and Food Chemistry*. 2010;58(7):3996–4000.

Kris-Etherton PM. AHA Science Advisory. Monounsaturated fatty acids and risk of cardiovascular disease. American Heart Association. Nutrition Committee. *Circulation*. 1999;100(11):1253–8.

Kuller LH. Dietary fat and chronic diseases: epidemiologic overview. *Journal of the American Dietetic Association*. 1997;97(Suppl 7):S9–15.

Kumar N, Goel N. Phenolic acids: natural versatile molecules with promising therapeutic applications. *Biotechnology Reports (Amst)*. 2019;24:e00370.

La Berge AF. How the ideology of low fat conquered America. *Journal of the History of Medicine and Allied Sciences*. 2008;63(2): 139–77.

Leyva-Soto A, Chavez-Santoscoy RA, Lara-Jacobo LR, et al. Daily consumption of chocolate rich in flavonoids decreases cellular genotoxicity and improves biochemical parameters of lipid and glucose metabolism. *Molecules*. 2018;23(9):2220.

Liu AG, Ford NA, Hu FB, et al. A healthy approach to dietary fats: understanding the science and taking action to reduce consumer confusion. *Nutrition Journal*. 2017;16(1):53.

Lv X, Zhao S, Ning Z, et al. Citrus fruits as a treasure trove of active natural metabolites that potentially provide benefits for human health. *Chemistry Central Journal*. 2015;9:68.

Malhotra A, Redberg RF, Meier P. Saturated fat does not clog the arteries: coronary heart disease is a chronic inflammatory condition, the risk of which can be effectively reduced from healthy lifestyle interventions. *British Journal of Sports Medicine*. 2017;51(15):1111–2.

Masters RC, Liese AD, Haffner SM, et al. Whole and refined grain intakes are related to inflammatory protein concentrations in human plasma. *Journal of Nutrition*. 2010;140(3):587–94.

Mazza G, Kay CD, Cottrell T, et al. Absorption of anthocyanins from blueberries and serum antioxidant status in human subjects. *Journal of Agricultural and Food Chemistry*. 2002;50(26):7731–7.

Medeiros-de-Moraes IM, Gonçalves-de-Albuquerque CF, Kurz ARM, et al. Omega-9 oleic acid, the main compound of olive oil, mitigates inflammation during experimental sepsis. *Oxidative Medicine and Cellular Longevity*. 2018;2018:6053492.

Menendez JA, Lupu R. Mediterranean dietary traditions for the molecular treatment of human cancer:

anti-oncogenic actions of the main olive oil's mono-unsaturated fatty acid oleic acid (18:1n-9). *Current Pharmaceutical Biotechnology.* 2006;7(6):495–502.

Menendez JA, Vellon L, Colomer R, et al. Oleic acid, the main monounsaturated fatty acid of olive oil, suppresses Her-2/neu (erbB-2) expression and synergistically enhances the growth inhibitory effects of trastuzumab (Herceptin) in breast cancer cells with Her-2/neu oncogene amplification. *Annals of Oncology.* 2005;16(3):359–71.

Miller MG, Shukitt-Hale B. Berry fruit enhances beneficial signaling in the brain. *Journal of Agricultural and Food Chemistry.* 2012;60(23):5709–15.

Moran NE, Johnson EJ. Closer to clarity on the effect of lipid consumption on fat-soluble vitamin and carotenoid absorption: do we need to close in further? *American Journal of Clinical Nutrition.* 2017;106(4):969–70.

Moreno-Indias I, Sánchez-Alcoholado L, Pérez-Martínez P, et al. Red wine polyphenols modulate fecal microbiota and reduce markers of the metabolic syndrome in obese patients. *Food and Function.* 2016;7(4):1775–87.

Nadeem HR, Akhtar, S, Ismail T, et al. Heterocyclic aromatic amines in meat: formation, isolation, risk assessment, and inhibitory effect of plant extracts. *Foods.* 2021;10:1466.

Orsavova J, Misurcova L, Ambrozova JV, et al. Fatty acids composition of vegetable oils and its contribution to dietary energy intake and dependence of cardiovascular mortality on dietary intake of fatty acids. *International Journal of Molecular Science.* 2015;16(6):12871–90.

Osterdahl BG. Volatile nitrosamines in foods on the Swedish market and estimation of their daily intake. *Food Additives and Contaminants.* 1988;5(4):587–95.

Rodríguez-García C, Sánchez-Quesada C, Toledo E, et al. Naturally lignan-rich foods: a dietary tool for health promotion? *Molecules.* 2019;24(5):917.

Rostami A, Khalili M, Haghighat N, et al. High-cocoa polyphenol-rich chocolate improves blood pressure in patients with diabetes and hypertension. *ARYA Atherosclerosis.* 2015;11(1):21–9.

Simopoulos AP. The importance of the ratio of omega-6/omega-3 essential fatty acids. *Biomedical Pharmacotherapy.* 2002;56(8):365–79.

Smit LA, Baylin A, Campos H. Conjugated linoleic acid in adipose tissue and risk of myocardial infarction. *American Journal of Clinical Nutrition.* 2010;92(1):34–40.

Sun Y, Qin H, Zhang H, et al. Fisetin inhibits inflammation and induces autophagy by mediating PI3K/AKT/mTOR signaling in LPS-induced RAW264.7 cells. *Food & Nutrition Research.* 2021;65:10.

Syed DN, Adhami VM, Khan MI, et al. Inhibition of Akt/mTOR signaling by the dietary flavonoid fisetin. *Anticancer Agents in Medicinal Chemistry.* 2013;13(7):995–1001.

Taylor RS, Ashton KE, Moxham T, et al. Reduced dietary salt for the prevention of cardiovascular disease: a meta-analysis of randomized controlled trials (Cochrane review). *American Journal of Hypertension.* 2011;24(8):843–53.

Torabian S, Haddad E, Rajaram S, et al. Acute effect of nut consumption on plasma total polyphenols, antioxidant capacity and lipid peroxidation. *Journal of Human Nutrition and Dietetics.* 2009;22(1):64–71.

Vigar V, Myers S, Oliver C, et al. A systematic review of organic versus conventional food consumption: is there a measurable benefit on human health? *Nutrients.* 2020;12(1):7.

Watras AC, Buchholz AC, Close RN, et al. The role of conjugated linoleic acid in reducing body fat and preventing holiday weight gain. *International Journal of Obesity (Lond).* 2007;31(3):481–7.

Wolfe KL, Kang X, He X, et al. Cellular antioxidant activity of common fruits. *Journal of Agricultural and Food Chemistry.* 2008;56(18):8418–26.

Wongmaneepratip W, Na Jom K, Vangnai K. Inhibitory effects of dietary antioxidants on the formation of carcinogenic polycyclic aromatic hydrocarbons in grilled pork. *Asian-Australasian Journal of Animal Science.* 2019;32(8):1205–10.

Worthington V. Nutritional quality of organic versus conventional fruits, vegetables, and grains. *The Journal of Alternative and Complementary Medicine.* 2001;7(2):161–73.

Zhang C, Adamos C, Oh MJ, et al. oxLDL induces endothelial cell proliferation via Rho/ROCK/Akt/p27[kip1] signaling: opposite effects of oxLDL and cholesterol loading. *American Journal of Physiology Cell Physiology.* 2017;313(3):C340–51.

Zhong VW, Van Horn L, Greenland P, et al. Associations of processed meat, unprocessed red meat, poultry, or fish intake with incident cardiovascular disease and all-cause mortality. *JAMA Internal Medicine.* 2020;180(4):503–12.

■ CHAPTER 6

Adamu B, Sani MU, Abdu A. Physical exercise and health: a review. *Nigerian Journal of Medicine.* 2006; 15(3):190–6.

Behm DG, Blazevich AJ, Kay AD, et al. Acute effects of muscle stretching on physical performance, range of motion, and injury incidence in healthy active individuals: a systematic review. *Applied Physiology, Nutrition, and Metabolism.* 2016;41(1):1–11.

Bird SR, Hawley JA. Update on the effects of physical activity on insulin sensitivity in humans. *BMJ Open Sport & Exercise Medicine.* 2017;2(1):e000143.

Casaletto K, Ramos-Miguel A, VandeBunte A, et al. Late-life physical activity relates to brain tissue synaptic integrity markers in older adults. *Alzheimer's & Dementia.* 2021;1–13.

Cortell-Tormo JM, Sánchez PT, Chulvi-Medrano I, et al. Effects of functional resistance training on fitness and quality of life in females with chronic nonspecific low-back pain. *Journal of Back and Musculoskeletal Rehabilitation.* 2018;31(1):95–105.

da Silva LA, Tortelli L, Motta J, et al. Effects of aquatic exercise on mental health, functional autonomy and oxidative stress in depressed elderly individuals: a randomized clinical trial. *Clinics (Sao Paulo).* 2019;74:e322.

da Silveira MP, da Silva Fagundes KK, Bizuti MR, et al. Physical exercise as a tool to help the immune system against COVID-19: an integrative review of the current literature. *Clinical and Experimental Medicine.* 2021;21(1):15–28.

Dorling J, Broom DR, Burns SF, et al. Acute and chronic effects of exercise on appetite, energy intake, and appetite-related hormones: the modulating effect of adiposity, sex, and habitual physical activity. *Nutrients.* 2018;10(9):1140.

Ferreira RM, Alves W, de Lima TA, et al. The effect of resistance training on the anxiety symptoms and quality of life in elderly people with Parkinson's disease: a randomized controlled trial. *Arq Neuropsiquiart.* 2018;76(8):499–506.

Fielding RA, Rejeski WJ, Blair S, et al. The Lifestyle Interventions and Independence for Elders Study: design and methods. *Journals of Gerontology Series A: Biological Science and Medical Sciences.* 2011;66(11):1226–37.

Flack KD, Hays HM, Moreland J, et al. Exercise for weight loss: further evaluating energy compensation with exercise. *Medicine and Science in Sports and Exercise.* 2020;52(11):2466–75.

Flockhart M, Nilsson LC, Tais S, et al. Excessive exercise training causes mitochondrial function impairment and decreases glucose tolerance in healthy volunteers. *Cell Metabolism.* 2021;33(5):957–70.

Garatachea N, Pareja-Galeano H, Sanchis-Gomar F, et al. Exercise attenuates the major hallmarks of aging. *Rejuvenation Research.* 2015;18(1):57–89.

Gordon BR, McDowell CP, Lyons M, et al. Resistance exercise training among young adults with analogue generalized anxiety disorder. *Journal of Affective Disorders.* 2021;281:153–9.

Hallgren M, Kraepelien M, Öjehagebn A, et al. Physical exercise and internet-based cognitive-behavioural therapy in the treatment of depression: randomised controlled trial. *British Journal of Psychiatry.* 2015;207(3):227–34.

Health Quality Ontario. Structured education and neuromuscular exercise program for hip and/or knee osteoarthritis: A Health Technology Assessment. *Ontario Health Technology Assessment Services.* 2018;18(8):1–110.

Henriksson M, Wall A, Nyberg J, et al. Effects of exercise on symptoms of anxiety in primary care patients: a randomized controlled trial. *Journal of Affective Disorders.* 2022;297:26.

Laker RC, Drake JC, Wilson RJ, *et al.* Ampk phosphorylation of Ulk1 is required for targeting of mitochondria to lysosomes in exercise-induced mitophagy. *Nature Communications.* 2017;8:548.

Lakoski SG, Willis, BL, Barlow CE, et al. Midlife cardiorespiratory fitness, incident cancer, and survival after cancer in men. The Cooper Center Longevity Study. *JAMA Oncology.* 2015;1(2):231–7.

Li G, Li J, Gao F. Exercise and cardiovascular protection. *Advances in Experimental Medicine and Biology.* 2020;1228:205–16.

Liberman K, Forti LN, Beyer I, et al. The effects of exercise on muscle strength, body composition, physical functioning, and the inflammatory profile of older adults: a systematic review. *Current Opinions in Clinical Nutrition and Metabolic Care*. 2017;20(1):30–53.

Mavros Y, Gates N, Wilson GC, et al. Mediation of cognitive function improvements by strength gains after resistance training in older adults with mild cognitive impairment: outcomes of the study of mental and resistance training. *Journal of the American Geriatric Society*. 2017;65(3):550–9.

Mazzilli KM, Matthews CE, Salerno EA, et al. Weight training and risk of 10 common types of cancer. *Medicine and Science in Sports and Exercise*. 2019;51(9):1845–51.

Minihan A, Patel A, Flanders W, et al. Proportion of cancer cases attributable to physical inactivity by US state, 2013–2016. *Medicine & Science in Sports & Exercise*. 2022;54(3):417–23.

Ramakrishnan R, Doherty A, Smith-Byrne K, et al. Accelerometer measured physical activity and the incidence of cardiovascular disease: evidence from the UK Biobank cohort study. *PLOS Medicine*. 2021;18(9):e1003809.

Moraes HS, Silveira HS, Oliveira NA, et al. Is strength training as effective as aerobic training for depression in older adults? A randomized controlled trial. *Neuropsychobiology*. 2020;79(2):141–9.

Nawrocka A, Polechonski J, Garbaciak W, et al. Functional fitness and quality of life among women over 60 years of age depending on their level of objectively measured physical activity. *International Journal of Environmental Research and Public Health*. 2019;16(6):972.

Nicol LM, Rowlands DS, Fazakerly R, et al. Curcumin supplementation likely attenuates delayed onset muscle soreness (DOMS). *European Journal of Applied Physiology*. 2015;115(8):1769–77.

Peterson NE, Osterloh KD, Graff MN. Exercises for older adults with knee and hip pain. *The Journal for Nurse Practitioners*. 2019;15(4):263–7.

Rundqvist H, Veliça P, Barbieri L, et al. Cytotoxic T-cells mediate exercise-induced reductions in tumor growth. *Elife*. 2020;9:e59996.

Rynecki ND, Siracuse BL, Ippolito JA, et al. Injuries sustained during high intensity interval training: are modern fitness trends contributing to increased injury rates? *Journal of Sports Medicine & Physical Fitness*. 2019;59(7):1206–12.

Simpson RJ, Kunz H, Agha N, et al. Exercise and the regulation of immune functions. *Progress in Molecular Biology and Translational Science*. 2015;135:355–80.

Tanabe Y, Chino K, Sagayama H, et al. Effective timing of curcumin ingestion to attenuate eccentric exercise-induced muscle soreness in men. *Journal of Nutritional Science and Vitaminology (Tokyo)*. 2019;65(1):82–9.

Wedell-Neergaard A, Lehrskov L, Christensen RH, et al. Exercise-induced changes in visceral adipose tissue mass are regulated by il-6 signaling: a randomized controlled trial. *Cell Metabolism*. 2019;29(4):844–55.e3.

Xirouchaki CE, Jia Y, McGrath MJ, et al. Skeletal muscle NOX4 is required for adaptive responses that prevent insulin resistance. *Science Advances*. 2021;7(51):eabl4988.

Yamada M, Nishiguchi S, Fukutani N, et al. Mail-based intervention for sarcopenia prevention increased anabolic hormone and skeletal muscle mass in community-dwelling Japanese older adults: the INE (Intervention by Nutrition and Exercise) Study. *Journal of the American Medical Director's Association*. 2015;16(8):654–60.

CHAPTER 7

Abbasi B, Kimiagar M, Sadeghniiat K, et al. The effect of magnesium supplementation on primary insomnia in elderly: a double-blind placebo-controlled clinical trial. *Journal of Research in Medical Sciences*. 2012;17(12):1161–9.

Aguirre CC. Sleep deprivation: a mind-body approach. *Current Options in Pulmonary Medicine*. 2016;22(6):583–8.

Asgari Mehrabadi M, Azimi I, Sarhaddi F, et al. Sleep tracking of a commercially available smart ring and smartwatch against medical-grade actigraphy in everyday settings: instrument validation study. *JMIR Mhealth Uhealth*. 2020;8(10):e20465.

Beattie L, Kyle SD, Espie CA, et al. Social interactions, emotion and sleep: a systematic review and research agenda. *Sleep Medicine Review*. 2015;24:83–100.

"Brain Basics: Understanding Sleep." National Institute of Neurological Disorders and Stroke. 2022. https://www.ninds.nih.gov/Disorders/Patient-Caregiver-Education/Understanding -Sleep.

Burkhart K, Phelps JR. Amber lenses to block blue light and improve sleep: a randomized trial. *Chronobiology International*. 2009;26(8):1602–12.

Buysse DJ. Insomnia. *JAMA*. 2013;309(7):706–16.

Cases J, Ibarra A, Feuillère N, et al. Pilot trial of *Melissa officinalis* L. leaf extract in the treatment of volunteers suffering from mild-to-moderate anxiety disorders and sleep disturbances. *Mediterranean Journal of Nutrition and Metabolism*. 2010;4(3):211–8.

Chandharakool S, Koomhin P, Sinlapasorn J, et al. Effects of tangerine essential oil on brain waves, moods, and sleep onset latency. *Molecules*. 2020;25(20):4865.

Chang A, Aeschbach D, Duffy LF, et al. Evening use of light-emitting eReaders negatively affects sleep, circadian timing, and next morning alertness. *PNAS*. 2014;112(4):1232–7.

Cousins JN, Fernández G. The impact of sleep deprivation on declarative memory. *Progress in Brain Research*. 2019;246:27–53.

Covassin N, Singh P, McCrady-Spitzer SK, et al. Effects of experimental sleep restriction on energy intake, energy expenditure, and visceral obesity. *Journal of the American College of Cardiology*. 2022;79(13):1254–65.

Dorrian J, Centofanti S, Smith A, et al. Self-regulation and social behavior during sleep deprivation. *Progress in Brain Research*. 2019;246:73–110.

Drugs and Lactation Database (LactMed) [Internet]. "Lavender." Bethesda (MD): National Library of Medicine (US). 2022.

Grifantini K. Tracking sleep to optimize health. *IEEE Pulse*. 2020;11(5):12–6.

Grubb S, Lauritzen M. Deep sleep drives brain fluid oscillations. *Science*. 2019;366(6465):572–3.

Guadagna S, Barattini DF, Rosu S, et al. Plant Extracts for sleep disturbances: a systematic review. *Evidenced-Based Complementary and Alternative Medicine*. 2020;2020:3792390.

Held K, Antonijevic IA, Künzel H, et al. Oral Mg2+ supplementation reverses age-related neuroendocrine and sleep EEG changes in humans. *Pharmacopsychiatry*. 2002;35(4):135–43.

Kaur H, Spurling BC, Bollu PC. "Chronic Insomnia." In: StatPearls [Internet]. Treasure Island (FL): StatPearls Publishing. 2022.

Kennedy DO, Little W, Scholey AB. Attenuation of laboratory-induced stress in humans after acute administration of *Melissa officinalis* (Lemon Balm). *Psychosomatic Medicine*. 2004;66(4):607–13.

Kim J, Lee SL, Kang I, et al. Natural products from single plants as sleep aids: a systematic review. *Journal of Medicinal Food*. 2018;21(5):433–44.

Krittanawong C, Tunhasiriwet A, Wang Z, et al. Association between short and long sleep durations and cardiovascular outcomes: a systematic review and meta-analysis. *European Heart Journal Acute Cardiovascular Care*. 2019;8(8):762–70.

Li J, Vitiello MV, Gooneratne NS. Sleep in normal aging. *Sleep Medicine Clinics*. 2018;13(1):1–11.

Lin J, Suurna M. Sleep apnea and sleep-disordered breathing. *Otolaryngologic Clinics of North America*. 2018;51(4):827–33.

Nguyen V, George T, Brewster GS. Insomnia in older adults. *Current Geriatrics Reports*. 2019;8(4):271–90.

Oh CM, Kim HY, Na HK, et al. The effect of anxiety and depression on sleep quality of individuals with high risk for insomnia: a population-based study. *Frontiers in Neurology*. 2019;10:849.

Okuro M, Morimoto S. Sleep apnea in the elderly. *Current Opinion in Psychiatry*. 2014;27(6):472–7.

Olivier B, Rakotoarison C, Harris R. Ravintsara vs ravensara a taxonomic clarification. *International Journal of Aromatherapy*. 2001;11(1):4–7.

Peuhkuri K, Sihvola N, Korpela R. Dietary factors and fluctuating levels of melatonin. *Food and Nutrition Research*. 2012;56.

Poleszak E. Benzodiazepine/GABA(A) receptors are involved in magnesium-induced anxiolytic-like behavior in mice. *Pharmacology Reports*. 2008;60(4):483–9.

Rasch B, Born J. About sleep's role in memory. *Physiological Reviews*. 2013;93(2):681–766.

"Sleep Statistics." The Sleep Foundation. https://www.sleepfoundation.org/how-sleep-works/sleep-facts-statistics.

Stuck BA, Hofauer B. The diagnosis and treatment of snoring in adults. *Dtsch Arztebl Int*. 2019;116(48):817–24.

Ulfberg J, Fenton G. Effect of Breathe Right nasal strip on snoring. *Rhinology*. 1997;35(2):50–2.

Voss P, Thomas ME, Cisneros-Franco JM, et al. Dynamic brains and the changing rules of neuroplasticity: Implications for learning and recovery. *Frontiers in Psychology*. 2017;8:1657.

Xu J, Niu YX, Piao XM, et al. Effect of acupuncture on blood oxygen saturation in patients of obstructive sleep apnea-hypopnea syndrome. *Zhongguo Zhen Jiu*. 2009;29(1):84–6.

Yaremchuk K. Why and when to treat snoring. *Otolaryngological Clinics of North America*. 2020;53(3):351–65.

■ CHAPTER 8

Aalbers S, Fusar-Poli L, Freeman RE, et al. Music therapy for depression. *Cochrane Database Systems Review*. 2017;11(11):CD004517.

Anghelescu I, Edwards D, Seifritz E, et al. Stress management and the role of *Rhodiola rosea*: a review. *International Journal of Psychiatry in Clinical Practice*. 2018;22(4):242–52.

Assadi SN. What are the effects of psychological stress and physical work on blood lipid profiles? *Medicine (Baltimore)*. 2017;96(18):e6816.

Cain CD. The effects of prayer as a coping strategy for nurses. *Journal of Paranesthesia Nurses*. 2019;34(6):1187–95.

Chandrasekhar K, Kapoor J, Anishetty S. A prospective, randomized double-blind, placebo-controlled study of safety and efficacy of a high-concentration full-spectrum extract of ashwagandha root in reducing stress and anxiety in adults. *Indian Journal of Psychological Medicine*. 2012;34(3):255–62.

Chu B, Marwaha K, Sanvictores T, et al. "Physiology, Stress Reaction." In: StatPearls [Internet]. Treasure Island (FL): StatPearls Publishing. 2022.

Colori S. Journaling as therapy. *Schizophrenia Bulletin*. 2018;44(2):226–8.

Dar T, Radfar A, Abohashem S, et al. Psychosocial stress and cardiovascular disease. *Current Treatment Options in Cardiovascular Medicine*. 2019;21(5):23.

Dias P, Pedro L, Pereira O, et al. Aromatherapy in the control of stress and anxiety. *Alternative & Integrative Medicine*. 2017;6:1–5.

Ebrahimi H, Mardani A, Basirinezhad MH, et al. The effects of Lavender and Chamomile essential oil inhalation aromatherapy on depression, anxiety and stress in older community-dwelling people: a randomized controlled trial. *Explore (NY)*. 2022;18(3):272–8.

Espinosa-Garcia C, Zeleke H, Rojas A. Impact of stress on epilepsy: focus on neuroinflammation-A mini review. *International Journal of Molecular Science*. 2021;22(8):4061.

Fiksdal A, Hanlin L, Kuras Y, et al. Associations between symptoms of depression and anxiety and cortisol responses to and recovery from acute stress. *Psychoneuroendocrinology*. 2019;102:44–52.

Foster JA, Rinaman L, Cryan JF. Stress & the gut-brain axis: regulation by the microbiome. *Neurobiology & Stress*. 2017;7:124–36.

Geng S, Yang L, Cheng F, et al. Gut microbiota are associated with psychological stress-induced defections in intestinal and blood-brain barriers. *Frontiers in Microbiology*. 2020;10:3067.

Goodman AM, Allendorfer JB, Heyse H, et al. Neural response to stress and perceived stress differ in patients with left temporal lobe epilepsy. *Human Brain Mapping*. 2019;40(12):3415–30.

Gordon AM, Mendes WB. A large-scale study of stress, emotions, and blood pressure in daily life using a digital platform. *PNAS*. 2021;118(31):e2105573118.

Hagström E, Norlund F, Stebbins A, et al. Psychosocial stress and major cardiovascular events in patients with stable coronary heart disease. *Journal of Internal Medicine*. 2018;283(1):83–92.

Haller J, Krecsak L, Zámbori J. Double-blind placebo controlled trial of the anxiolytic effects of a standardized Echinacea extract. *Phytotherapy Research*. 2020;34(3):660–8.

Harris ML, Oldmeadow C, Hure A, et al. Stress increases the risk of type 2 diabetes onset in women: a 12-year longitudinal study using causal modelling. *PLOS ONE*. 2017;12(2):e0172126.

Hoge EA, Bui E, Marques L, et al. Randomized controlled trial of mindfulness meditation for generalized anxiety disorder: effects on anxiety and stress reactivity. *Journal of Clinical Psychiatry*. 2013;74(8):786–92.

Huang F, Chien D, Chung U. Effects of hatha yoga on stress in middle-aged women. *Journal of Nursing Research*. 2013;21(1):59–66.

Infante JR, Torres-Avisbal M, Pinel P, et al. Catecholamine levels in practitioners of the transcendental meditation technique. *Physiology & Behavior.* 2001;72(1-2):141–6.

Jevning R, Wilson AF, Davidson JM. Adrenocortical activity during meditation. *Hormones & Behavior.* 1978;10(1):54–60.

Justice NJ. The relationship between stress and Alzheimer's disease. *Neurobiology of Stress.* 2018;8:127–33.

Karin O, Raz M, Tendler A, et al. A new model for the HPA axis explains dysregulation of stress hormones on the timescale of weeks. *Molecular Systems Biology.* 2020;16(7):e9510.

Lai HL, Li YM. The effect of music on biochemical markers and self-perceived stress among first-line nurses: a randomized controlled crossover trial. *Journal of Advanced Nursing.* 2011;67(11):2414–24.

Li L, Li X, Zhou W, et al. Acute psychological stress results in the rapid development of insulin resistance. *Journal of Endocrinology.* 2013;217(2):175–84.

Linnemann A, Ditzen B, Strahler J, et al. Music listening as a means of stress reduction in daily life. *Psychoneuroendocrinology.* 2015;60:82–90.

Lopresti A, Smith SJ, Malvi H, et al. An investigation into the stress-relieving and pharmacological actions of an ashwagandha (*Withania somnifera*) extract. *Medicine.* 2019;98(37):e17186.

Ma GP, Zheng Q, Xu MB, et al. *Rhodiola rosea* L. improves learning and memory function: preclinical evidence and possible mechanisms. *Frontiers in Pharmacology.* 2018;9:1415.

"Meditation and Mindfulness: What You Need To Know." National Center for Complementary and Integrative Health. 2022. https://www.nccih.nih.gov/health/meditation-in-depth.

Meng L, Zhang Y, Luo Y, et al. Chronic stress a potential suspect zero of atherosclerosis: a systematic review. *Frontiers in Cardiovascular Medicine.* 2021;8:738654.

Morey JN, Boggero IA, Scott AB, et al. Current directions in stress and human immune function. *Current Opinions in Psychology.* 2015;5:13–7.

Ozgundondu B, Gok Metin Z. Effects of progressive muscle relaxation combined with music on stress, fatigue, and coping styles among intensive care nurses. *Intensive Critical Care Nursing.* 2019;54:54–63.

Peavy GM, Jacobson MW, Salmon DP, et al. The influence of chronic stress on dementia-related diagnostic change in older adults. *Alzheimer's Disease and Associated Disorders.* 2012;26(3):260–6.

Peña-Bautista C, Casas-Fernández E, Vento M, et al. Stress and neurodegeneration. *International Journal of Clinical Chemistry.* 2020;503:163–8.

Pellissier S, Bonaz B. The place of stress and emotions in the irritable bowel syndrome. *Vitamins & Hormones.* 2017;103:327–54.

Pouwer F, Kupper N, Adriaanse MC. Does emotional stress cause type 2 diabetes mellitus? A review from the European Depression in Diabetes (EDID) Research Consortium. *Discovery Medicine.* 2010;9(45):112–8.

Salimpoor V, Benovoy M, Larcher K, *et al.* Anatomically distinct dopamine release during anticipation and experience of peak emotion to music. *Nature Neuroscience.* 2011;14:257–62.

Salve J, Pate S, Debnath K, et al. Adaptogenic and anxiolytic effects of ashwagandha root extract in healthy adults: a double-blind, randomized, placebo-controlled clinical study. *Cureus.* 2019;11(12):e6466.

Scott SB, Graham-Engeland JE, Engeland CG, et al. The effects of stress on cognitive aging, physiology and emotion (ESCAPE) project. *BMC Psychiatry.* 2015;15:146.

Seiler A, Fagundes CP, Christian LM. The impact of everyday stressors on the immune system and health. *Stress Challenges and Immunity in Space.* 2020;71–92.

Sharma R, Gupta D, Mehrotra R, et al. Psychobiotics: the next-generation probiotics for the brain. *Current Microbiology.* 2021;78(2):449–63.

Shohani M, Badfar G, Nasirkandy MP, et al. The effect of yoga on stress, anxiety, and depression in women. *International Journal of Preventive Medicine.* 2018;9:21.

Smith SM, Vale WW. The role of the hypothalamic-pituitary-adrenal axis in neuroendocrine responses to stress. *Dialogues in Clinical Neuroscience.* 2006;8(4):383–95.

Song H, Fang F, Arnberg FK, et al. Stress related disorders and risk of cardiovascular disease: population based, sibling controlled cohort study. *BMJ.* 2019;365.

Stephens MA, Wand G. Stress and the HPA axis: role of glucocorticoids in alcohol dependence. *Alcohol Research.* 2012;34(4):468–83.

Sun Y, Li L, Xie R, et al. Stress triggers flare of inflammatory bowel disease in children and adults. *Frontiers in Pediatrics*. 2019;7:432.

Sussams R, Schlotz W, Clough Z, et al. Psychological stress, cognitive decline and the development of dementia in amnestic mild cognitive impairment. *Scientific Reports*. 2020;10:3618.

Swinkels WA, Engelsman M, Kasteleijn-Nolst Trenité DG, et al. Influence of an evacuation in February 1995 in The Netherlands on the seizure frequency in patients with epilepsy: a controlled study. *Epilepsia*. 1998;39(11):1203–7.

Turner L, Galante J, Vainre M, et al. Immune dysregulation among students exposed to exam stress and its mitigation by mindfulness training: findings from an exploratory randomised trial. *Scientific Reports*. 2020;10:5812.

Umbrello M, Sorrenti T, Mistraletti G, et al. Music therapy reduces stress and anxiety in critically ill patients: a systematic review of randomized clinical trials. *Minerva Anestesiologica*. 2019;85(8):886–98.

"What Happens to the Brain in Alzheimer's Disease?" National Institute on Aging. 2017. https://www.nia.nih.gov/health/what-happens-brain-alzheimers-disease.

Zollars I, Poirier TI, Pailden J. Effects of mindfulness meditation on mindfulness, mental well-being, and perceived stress. *Currents in Pharmacy Teaching & Learning*. 2019;11(10):1022–8.

■ CHAPTER 9

Abe Y, Hashimoto S, Horie T. Curcumin inhibition of inflammatory cytokine production by human peripheral blood monocytes and alveolar macrophages. *Pharmacology Research*. 1999;38(1):41–7.

Age-Related Eye Disease Study Research Group. A randomized, placebo-controlled, clinical trial of high-dose supplementation with vitamins C and E, beta carotene, and zinc for age-related macular degeneration and vision loss: AREDS report no. 8. *Archives of Ophthalmology*. 2001;119:1417–36.

Ak T, Gülcin I. Antioxidant and radical scavenging properties of curcumin. *Chemical-Biological Interactions*. 2008;174(1):27–37.

Alanzi A, Honkala S, Honkala E, et al. Effect of *Lactobacillus rhamnosus* and *Bifidobacterium lactis* on gingival health, dental plaque, and periodontopathogens in adolescents: a randomised placebo-controlled clinical trial. *Beneficial Microbes*. 2018;9(4):593–602.

Albracht-Schulte K, Kalupahana NS, Ramalingam L, et al. Omega-3 fatty acids in obesity and metabolic syndrome: a mechanistic update. *Journal of Nutritional Biochemistry*. 2018;58:1–16.

Anand P, Kunnumakkara AB, Newman RA, et al. Bioavailability of curcumin: problems and promises. *Molecular Pharmaceutics*. 2007;4(6):807–18.

Antony B, Merina B, Iyer VS, et al. A pilot crossover study to evaluate human oral bioavailability of BCM-95CG (Biocurcumax), a novel bioenhanced preparation of curcumin. *Indian Journal Pharmaceutical Sciences*. 2008;70(4):445–9.

Bae JM. Prophylactic efficacy of probiotics on travelers' diarrhea: an adaptive meta-analysis of randomized controlled trials. *Epidemiological Health*. 2018;40:e2018043.

Bailey RL, Fakhouri TH, Park Y, et al. Multivitamin-mineral use is associated with reduced risk of cardiovascular disease mortality among women in the United States. *Journal of Nutrition*. 2015;145(3):572–8.

Bailey RL, Gahche JJ, Lentino CV, et al. Dietary supplement use in the United States, 2003–2006. *Journal of Nutrition*. 2011;141(2):261–6.

Baker LD, Rapp SR, Shumaker SA, et al. Design and baseline characteristics of the cocoa supplement and multivitamin outcomes study for the Mind: COSMOS-Mind. *Contemporary Clinical Trials*. 2019;83:57–63.

Balvers MG, Brouwer-Brolsma EM, Endenburg S, et al. Recommended intakes of vitamin D to optimise health, associated circulating 25-hydroxyvitamin D concentrations, and dosing regimens to treat deficiency: workshop report and overview of current literature. *Journal of Nutritional Science*. 2015;4:e23.

Barreto FM, Colado Simão AN, Morimoto HK, et al. Beneficial effects of *Lactobacillus plantarum* on glycemia and homocysteine levels in postmenopausal women with metabolic syndrome. *Nutrition*. 2014;30(7–8):939–42.

Bathina S. Das UN. Brain-derived neurotrophic factor and its clinical implications. *Archives of Medical Science*. 2015;11(6):1164–78.

Behboudi-Gandevani S, Hariri FZ, Moghaddam-Banaem L. The effect of omega 3 fatty acid supplementation on premenstrual syndrome and health-related quality of life: a randomized clinical trial. *Journal of Psychosomatic Obstetrics and Gynaecology*. 2018;39(4):266–72.

Bernstein AM, Ding EL, Willett WC, et al. A meta-analysis shows that docosahexaenoic acid from algal oil reduces serum triglycerides and increases HDL-cholesterol and LDL-cholesterol in persons without coronary heart disease. *Journal of Nutrition*. 2012;142(1):99–104.

Bhardwaj RK, Glaeser H, Becquemont L, et al. Piperine, a major constituent of black pepper, inhibits human P-glycoprotein and CYP3A4. *Journal of Pharmacology & Experimental Therapeutics*. 2002;302(2):645–50.

Bianchi VE. Impact of nutrition on cardiovascular function. *Current Problems in Cardiology*. 2020;45(1):100391.

Blumberg JB, Bailey RL, Sesso HD, et al. The evolving role of multivitamin/multimineral supplement use among adults in the age of personalized nutrition. *Nutrients*. 2018;10:248.

Carroll D, Ring C, Suter M, et al. The effects of an oral multivitamin combination with calcium, magnesium, and zinc on psychological well-being in healthy young male volunteers: a double-blind placebo-controlled trial. *Psychopharmacology (Berl)*. 2000;150(2):220–5.

Chang YH, Becnel J, Trudo S. Effects of multivitamin-mineral supplementation on mental health among young adults (OR15-03-19). *Current Developments in Nutrition*. 2019;3(Suppl 1):nzz044.OR15-03-19.

Christen WG, Glynn RJ, Manson et al. Effects of multivitamin supplement on cataract and age-related macular degeneration in a randomized trial of male physicians. *Ophthalmology*. 2014;121(2):525–34.

Dobryniewski J, Szajda SD, Waszkiewicz N, et al. The gama-linolenic acid (GLA)—the therapeutic value. *Przegl Lek*. 2007;64:100–2.

Ekholm P, Virkki L, Ylinen M, et al. The effect of phytic acid and some natural chelating agents on the solubility of mineral elements in oat bran. *Food Chemistry*. 2003;80(2):165–70.

Eslick GD, Howe PRC, Smith C, et al. Benefits of fish oil supplementation in hyperlipidemia: a systematic review and meta-analysis. *International Journal of Cardiology*. 2009;136(1):4–16.

Fu YR, Yi ZJ, Pei JL, et al. Effects of *Bifidobacterium bifidum* on adaptive immune senescence in aging mice. *Microbiology and Immunology*. 2010;54(10):578–83.

Fuentes MC, Lajo T, Carrión JM, et al. Cholesterol-lowering efficacy of *Lactobacillus plantarum* CECT 7527, 7528 and 7529 in hypercholesterolaemic adults. *British Journal of Nutrition*. 2013;109(10):1866–72.

Ginty AT, Conklin SM. Short-term supplementation of acute long-chain omega-3 polyunsaturated fatty acids may alter depression status and decrease symptomology among young adults with depression: a preliminary randomized and placebo controlled trial. *Psychiatry Research*. 2015;229(1-2):485–9.

Giovannucci E, Stampfer MJ, Colditz GA, et al. Multivitamin use, folate, and colon cancer in women in the Nurses' Health Study. *Annals of Internal Medicine*. 1998;129(7):517–24.

Gioxari A, Kaliora AC, Marantidou F, et al. Intake of ω-3 polyunsaturated fatty acids in patients with rheumatoid arthritis: a systematic review and meta-analysis. *Nutrition*. 2018;45:114–24.e4.

Goel A, Kunnumakkara AB, Aggarwal BB. Curcumin as "Curecumin": from kitchen to clinic. *Biochemical Pharmacology*. 2008;75(4):787–809.

Gomi A, Iino T, Nonaka C, et al. Health benefits of fermented milk containing *Bifidobacterium bifidum* YIT 10347 on gastric symptoms in adults. *Journal of Dairy Science*. 2015;98(4):2277–83.

Grin PM, Kowalewska PM, Alhazzan W, et al. *Lactobacillus* for preventing recurrent urinary tract infections in women: meta-analysis. *Canadian Journal of Urology*. 2013;20(1):6607–14.

Haroyan A, Mukuchyan V, Mkrtchyan N, et al. Efficacy and safety of curcumin and its combination with boswellic acid in osteoarthritis: a comparative, randomized, double-blind, placebo-controlled study. *BMC Complementary and Alternative Medicine*. 2018;17:7.

Gröber U, Schmidt J, Kisters K. Magnesium in prevention and therapy. *Nutrients*. 2015;7(9):8199–226.

Halder M, Petsophonsakul P, Akbulut AC, et al. Vitamin K: double bonds beyond coagulation insights into differences between vitamin K1 and K2 in health and disease. *International Journal of Molecular Science*. 2019;20(4):896.

Harris E, Kirk J, Rowsell R, et al. The effect of multivitamin supplementation on mood and stress in healthy older men. *Human Psychopharmacology*. 2011;26(8):560–7.

Harris E, Macpherson H, Vitetta L, et al. Effects of a multivitamin, mineral and herbal supplement on cognition and blood biomarkers in older men: a randomised, placebo-controlled trial. *Human Psychopharmacology*. 2012;27(4):370–7.

Heintz-Buschart A, Wilmes P. Human gut microbiome: function matters. *Trends in Microbiology*. 2018;26(7):563–74.

Hilton E, Kolakowski P, Singer C, et al. Efficacy of *Lactobacillus* GG as a diarrheal preventive in travelers. *Journal of Travel Medicine*. 1997;4(1):41–3.

Holick MF. The vitamin D deficiency pandemic: Approaches for diagnosis, treatment and prevention. *Review of Endocrine & Metabolic Disorders*. 2017;18(2):153–65.

Holmquist C, Larsson S, Wolk A, et al. Multivitamin supplements are inversely associated with risk of myocardial infarction in men and women--Stockholm Heart Epidemiology Program (SHEEP). *Journal of Nutrition*. 2003;133(8):2650–4.

Horrobin DF. Essential fatty acid metabolism and its modification in atopic eczema. *American Journal of Clinical Nutrition*. 2000;71:367S–72S.

Huang HY, Caballero B, Chang S, et al. The efficacy and safety of multivitamin and mineral supplement use to prevent cancer and chronic disease in adults: a systematic review for a National Institutes of Health state-of-the-science conference. *Annals of Internal Medicine*. 2006;145(5):372–85.

Ikonte CJ, Mun JG, Reider CA, et al. Micronutrient inadequacy in short sleep: analysis of the NHANES 2005-2016. *Nutrients*. 2019;11(10):2335.

Innes JK, Calder PC. Omega-6 fatty acids and inflammation. *Prostaglandins, Leukotrienes, & Essential Fatty Acids*. 2018;132:41–8.

Jageitia GC, Rajanikant GK. Curcumin stimulates the antioxidant mechanisms in mouse skin exposed to fractionated γ-irradiation. *Antioxidants*. 2015;4:25–41.

Jazayeri S, Tehrani-Doost M, Keshavarz SA, et al. Comparison of therapeutic effects of omega-3 fatty acid eicosapentaenoic acid and fluoxetine, separately and in combination, in major depressive disorder. *Australian and New Zealand Journal of Psychiatry*. 2008;42(3):192–8.

Jiang H, Shi X, Fan Y, et al. Dietary omega-3 polyunsaturated fatty acids and fish intake and risk of age-related macular degeneration. *Clinical Nutrition*. 2021;40(12):5662–73.

Kaewarpai T, Thongboonkerd V. High-glucose-induced changes in macrophage secretome: regulation of immune response. *Molecular & Cellular Biochemistry*. 2019;452(1–2):51–62.

Kazmierczak-Siedlecka K, Daca A, Folwarski M, et al. The role of *Lactobacillus plantarum* 299v in supporting treatment of selected diseases. *Central European Journal of Immunology*. 2019;45(4):488–93.

Kaur D, Rasane P, Singh J, et al. Nutritional interventions for elderly and considerations for the development of geriatric foods. *Current Aging Science*. 2019;12(1):15–27.

Khan SU, Lone AN, Khan MS, et al. Effect of omega-3 fatty acids on cardiovascular outcomes: a systematic review and meta-analysis. *EClinicalMedicine*. 2021;38:100997.

Kim SW, Park KY, Kim B, et al. *Lactobacillus rhamnosus* GG improves insulin sensitivity and reduces adiposity in high-fat diet-fed mice through enhancement of adiponectin production. *Biochemical and Biophysical Research Communications*. 2013;431(2):25–63.

Kligler B, Cohrssen A. Probiotics. *American Family Physician*. 2008;78(9):1073–8.

Kruger MC, Horrobin DF. Calcium metabolism, osteoporosis and essential fatty acids: a review. *Progress in Lipid Research*. 1997;36(2–3):131–51.

Kulkarni SK, Bhutani MK, Bishnoi M. Antidepressant activity of curcumin: involvement of serotonin and dopamine system. *Psychopharmacoclogy*. 2008;201:435.

Lai HT, de Oliveira Otto MC, Lemaitre RN, et al. Serial circulating omega 3 polyunsaturated fatty acids and healthy ageing among older adults in the Cardiovascular Health Study: prospective cohort study. *BMJ*. 2018;363:k4067.

Lai B, Kapoor AK, Asthana OP, et al. Efficacy of curcumin in the management of chronic anterior uveitis. *Phytotherapy Research*. 1999;13(4):318–22.

Lee DE, Huh CS, Ra J, et al. Clinical evidence of effects of *Lactobacillus plantarum* HY7714 on skin aging: a randomized, double blind, placebo-controlled study. *Journal of Microbiology and Biotechnology.* 2015;25(12):2160–8.

Li X, Feng K, Li J, et al. Curcumin inhibits apoptosis of chondrocytes through activation ERK1/2 signaling pathways induced autophagy. *Nutrients.* 2017;9(4):414.

Lopresti AL. The effects of psychological and environmental stress on micronutrient concentrations in the body: a review of the evidence. *Advances in Nutrition.* 2020;11(1):103–12.

Manore, MM. Effect of physical activity on thiamine, riboflavin, and vitamin B-6 requirements. *American Journal of Clinical Nutrition.* 2000;72(2):598S–606S.

Mancuso C, Barone E. Curcumin in clinical practice: myth or reality? *Trends in Pharmacological Science.* 2009;30:333–4.

Martí Del Moral A, Fortique F. Omega-3 fatty acids and cognitive decline: a systematic review. *Nutrición Hospitalaria.* 2019;36(4):939–49.

Martinez JE, Kahana DD, Ghuman S, et al. Unhealthy lifestyle and gut dysbiosis: a better understanding of the effects of poor diet and nicotine on the intestinal microbiome. *Frontiers in Endocrinology. (Lausanne).* 2021;12:667066.

"Milestones in Microbiota Research." Nature.com. 2019. www.nature.com/immersive/d42859-019-00041-z/index.html.

Mishra S, Palanivelu K. The effect of curcumin (turmeric) on Alzheimer's disease: an overview. *Annals of Indian Academy of Neurology.* 2008;11(1):13–9.

Mohajeri MH, La Fata G, Steinert RE, et al. Relationship between the gut microbiome and brain function. *Nutrition Reviews.* 2018;76(7):481–96.

Mohn ES, Kern HJ, Saltzman E, et al. Evidence of drug-nutrient interactions with chronic use of commonly prescribed medications: an update. *Pharmaceutics.* 2018;10(1):36.

Multivitamin/mineral Supplements. National Institutes of Health Office of Dietary Supplements. 2022. https://ods.od.nih.gov/factsheets/MVMS-HealthProfessional.

Murphy RA, Devarshi PP, Ekimura S, et al. Long-chain omega-3 fatty acid serum concentrations across life stages in the USA: an analysis of NHANES 2011–2012. *BMJ Open.* 2021;11:e043301.

Näse L, Hatakka K, Savilahti E, et al. Effect of long-term consumption of a probiotic bacterium, *Lactobacillus rhamnosus* GG, in milk on dental caries and caries risk in children. *Caries Research.* 2001;35(6):412–20.

Nishimura M, Ohkawara T, Tetsuka K, et al. Effects of yogurt containing *Lactobacillus plantarum* HOKKAIDO on immune function and stress markers. *Journal of Traditional and Complementary Medicine.* 2015;6(3):275–80.

Olek A, Woynarowski M, Ahrén IL, et al. Efficacy and safety of *Lactobacillus plantarum* DSM 9843 (LP299V) in the prevention of antibiotic-associated gastrointestinal symptoms in children—randomized, double-blind, placebo-controlled study. *Journal of Pediatrics.* 2017;186:82–6.

Oliveira JM, Rondó PHC. Omega-3 fatty acids and hypertriglyceridemia in HIV-infected subjects on antiretroviral therapy: systematic review and meta-analysis. *HIV Clinical Trials.* 2011;12(5):268–74.

Omega-3 Fatty Acids. National Institutes of Health Office of Dietary Supplements. 2022. https://ods.od.nih.gov/factsheets/Omega3FattyAcids-HealthProfessional.

Ozdemir O. Various effects of different probiotic strains in allergic disorders: an update from laboratory and clinical data. *Clinical and Experimental Immunology.* 2010;160(3):295–304.

Park S, Kang J, Choi S, et al. Cholesterol-lowering effect of *Lactobacillus rhamnosus* BFE5264 and its influence on the gut microbiome and propionate level in a murine model. *PLOS ONE.* 2018;13(8):e0203150.

Parker HM, Johnson NA, Burdon CA, et al. Omega-3 supplementation and non-alcoholic fatty liver disease: a systematic review and meta-analysis. *Journal of Hepatology.* 2012;56(4):944–51.

Pipingas A, Camfield DA, Stough C, et al. Effects of multivitamin, mineral and herbal supplement on cognition in younger adults and the contribution of B group vitamins. *Human Psychopharmacology.* 2014;29(1):73–82.

Prasad S, Aggarwal BB. "Turmeric, the Golden Spice: From Traditional Medicine to Modern Medicine." *Herbal Medicine: Biomolecular and Clinical Aspects.* 2011. 2nd edition. Boca Raton (FL): CRC Press/Taylor & Francis; Chapter 13.

Ramel A, Martinez JA, Kiely M, et al. Moderate consumption of fatty fish reduces diastolic blood pressure in overweight and obese European young adults during energy restriction. *Nutrition.* 2010;26(2):168–74.

Ramirez-Tortosa M, Mesa MD, Aguilera CM, et al. Oral administration of a turmeric extract inhibits LDL oxidation and has hypocholesterolemic effects in rabbits with experimental atherosclerosis. *Atherosclerosis.* 2000;147(2):371–8.

Rautiainen S, Rist PM, Glynn RJ, et al. Multivitamin use and the risk of cardiovascular disease in men. *Journal of Nutrition.* 2016;146:1235–40.

Ren R, Liu J, Cheng G, et al. Vitamin K2 (Menaquinone-7) supplementation does not affect vitamin K-dependent coagulation factors activity in healthy individuals. *Medicine (Baltimore).* 2021;100(23):e26221.

Robinson JG, Ijioma N, Harris W. Omega-3 fatty acids and cognitive function in women. *Women's Health (Lond).* 2010;6(1):119–34.

Sanmukhani J, Satodia V, Trivedi J, et al. Efficacy and safety of curcumin in major depressive disorder: a randomized controlled trial. *Phytotherapy Research.* 2014;28(4):579–85.

Santos-Parker JR, Strahler TR, Bassett CJ, et al. Curcumin supplementation improves vascular endothelial function in healthy middle-aged and older adults by increasing nitric oxide bioavailability and reducing oxidative stress. *Aging (Albany NY).* 2017;9(1):187–208.

Sarraf P, Parohan M, Javanbakht MH, et al. Short-term curcumin supplementation enhances serum brain-derived neurotrophic factor in adult men and women: a systematic review and dose-response meta-analysis of randomized controlled trials. *Nutrition Research.* 2019;69:1–8.

Satokar VV, Cutfield WS, Cameron-Smith D, et al. Response to Bannenberg and Rice. *Nutrition Reviewer.* 2022;80(1):138–40.

Schurgers LJ, Teunissen KJ, Hamulyák K, et al. Vitamin K-containing dietary supplements: comparison of synthetic vitamin K1 and natto-derived menaquinone-7. *Blood.* 2007;109(8):3279–83.

Schwalfenberg GK. Vitamins K1 and K2: The emerging group of vitamins required for human health. *Journal of Nutrition and Metabolism.* 2017;2017:6254836.

Shah BG. Chelating agents and bioavailability of minerals. *Nutrition Research.* 1981;1(6):617–22.

Sharma P, Bhardwaj P, Singh R. Administration of *Lactobacillus casei* and *Bifidobacterium bifidum* ameliorated hyperglycemia, dyslipidemia, and oxidative stress in diabetic rats. *International Journal of Preventive Medicine.* 2016;7:102.

Shep D, Khanwelkar C, Gade P, et al. Safety and efficacy of curcumin versus diclofenac in knee osteoarthritis: a randomized open-label parallel-arm study. *Trials.* 2019;20(1):214.

Shi N, Li N, Duan X, et al. Interaction between the gut microbiome and mucosal immune system. *Military Medical Research.* 2017;4:14.

Shin SK, Ha T, McGregor RA, et al. Long-term curcumin administration protects against atherosclerosis via hepatic regulation of lipoprotein cholesterol metabolism. *Molecular Nutrition and Food Research.* 2011;55:182–40.

Sidhu M, van der Poorten D. The gut microbiome. *Australian Family Physician.* 2017;46(4):206–11.

Simopoulos AP. The importance of the omega-6/omega-3 fatty acid ratio in cardiovascular disease and other chronic diseases. *Experimental Biology and Medicine.* 2008;233(6):674–88.

Simopoulos AP. The importance of the ratio of omega-6/omega-3 essential fatty acids. *Biomed Pharmacother.* 2002;56(8):365–79.

Simopoulos AP. The omega-6/omega-3 fatty acid ratio: health implications. *OCL.* 2010;17(5):267–75.

Small GW, Siddarth P, Li Z, et al. Memory and brain amyloid and tau effects of a bioavailable form of curcumin in non-demented adults: a double-blind, placebo-controlled 18-month trial. *The American Journal of Geriatric Psychiatry.* 2018;26(3):266–77.

Smith FI, Atherton P, Reeds, DN, et al. Dietary omega-3 fatty acid supplementation increases the rate of muscle protein synthesis in older adults: a randomized controlled trial. *American Journal of Clinical Nutrition.* 2011;93(2):402–12.

Soleimani A, Zarrati Mojarrad M, Bahmani F, et al. Probiotic supplementation in diabetic hemodialysis patients has beneficial metabolic effects. *Kidney International.* 2017;91(2):435–42.

Stevenson C, Blaauw R, Fredericks E, et al. Randomized clinical trial: effect of *Lactobacillus plantarum* 299v on symptoms of irritable bowel syndrome. *Nutrition.* 2014;30(10):1151–7.

Strasser B, Geiger D, Schauer M, et al. Probiotic supplements beneficially affect tryptophan-kynurenine metabolism and reduce the incidence of upper respiratory tract infections in trained athletes: a randomized, double-blinded, placebo-controlled trial. *Nutrients*. 2016;8(11):752.

Su KP, Huang SY, Chiu CC, et al. Omega-3 fatty acids in major depressive disorder. A preliminary double-blind, placebo-controlled trial. *European Neuropsychopharmacology*. 2003;13(4):267–71.

Summers WK, Martin RL, Cunningham M, et al. Complex antioxidant blend improves memory in community-dwelling seniors. *Journal of Alzheimer's Disease*. 2010;19(2):429–39.

"Supporting Older Patients with Chronic Conditions." National Institute on Aging. 2017. www.nia .nih.gov/health/supporting-older-patients -chronic-conditions.

Suresh, P, Srinivasan, K. Influence of curcumin, capsaicin, and piperine on the rat liver drug-metabolizing enzyme system in vivo and in vitro. *Canadian Journal of Physiology and Pharmacology*. 2007;84:1259–65.

Szajewska H, Kołodziej M. Systematic review with meta-analysis: *Lactobacillus rhamnosus* GG in the prevention of antibiotic-associated diarrhoea in children and adults. *Alimentary Pharmacology & Therapeutics*. 2015;42(10):1149–57.

Takada Y, Bhardwaj A, Potdar P, et al. Nonsteroidal anti-inflammatory agents differ in their ability to suppress NF-kappB activation, inhibition of expression of cyclooxygenase-2 and cyclin D1, and abrogation of tumor cell proliferation. *Oncogene*. 2004;23(57):9247–58.

Tompkins TA, Mainville I, Arcand Y. The impact of meals on a probiotic during transit through a model of the human upper gastrointestinal tract. *Beneficial Microbes*. 2011;2(4):295–303.

Thota RN, Dias CB, Abbott KA, et al. Curcumin alleviates postprandial glycaemic response in healthy subjects: a cross-over, randomized controlled study. *Scientific Reports*. 2018;8(1):13679.

Tripkovic L, Lambert H, Hart K, et al. Comparison of vitamin D2 and vitamin D3 supplementation in raising serum 25-hydroxyvitamin D status: a systematic review and meta-analysis. *American Journal of Clinical Nutrition*. 2012;95(6):1357-64.

Urita Y, Goto M, Watanabe T, et al. Continuous consumption of fermented milk containing *Bifidobacterium bifidum* YIT 10347 improves gastrointestinal and psychological symptoms in patients with functional gastrointestinal disorders. *Bioscience of Microbiota Food and Health*. 2015;34(2):37–44.

Vallon V, Thomson SC. The tubular hypothesis of nephron filtration and diabetic kidney disease. *Nature Reviews Nephrology*. 2020;16(6):317–36.

Wang BG, Xu HB, Wei H, et al. Oral administration of *Bifidobacterium bifidum* for modulating microflora, acid and bile resistance, and physiological indices in mice. *Canadian Journal of Microbiology*. 2015;61(2):155–63.

Wang Q, Liang X, Wang L, et al. Effect of omega-3 fatty acids supplementation on endothelial function: a meta-analysis of randomized controlled trials. *Atherosclerosis*. 2012;221(2):536–43.

White E, Shannon JS, Patterson RE. Relationship between vitamin and calcium supplement use and colon cancer. *Cancer Epidemiology Biomarkers and Prevention*. 1997;6(10):769–74.

Wongcharoen W, Jai-aue S, Phrommintikul A, et al. Effects of curcuminoids on frequency of acute myocardial infarction after coronary artery bypass grafting. *The American Journal of Cardiology*. 2012;110(1):40–4.

Wongcharoen W, Phrommintikul A. The protective role of curcumin in cardiovascular diseases. *International Journal of Cardiology*. 2009;133:145–51.

Xu Q, Parks CG, DeRoo LA, et al. Multivitamin use and telomere length in women. *American Journal of Clinical Nutrition*. 2009;303:250–7.

Xu Y, Ku BS, Yao, HY, et al. The effects of curcumin on depressive-like behaviors in mice. *European Journal of Pharmacology*. 2005;518(1):40–6.

Yang H, Xun P, He K. Fish and fish oil intake in relation to risk of asthma: a systematic review and meta-analysis. *PLOS ONE*. 2013;8(11):e80048.

Zhao LQ, Li LM, Zhu H, et al. The effect of multivitamin/mineral supplements on age-related cataracts: a systematic review and meta-analysis. *Nutrients*. 2014;6(3):931–49.

Zhao Y, Wang Z. Gut microbiome and cardiovascular disease. *Current Opinions in Cardiology*. 2020;35(3):207–8.

■ CHAPTER 10

Alarim RA, Alasmre FA, Alotaibi HA, et al. Effects of the ketogenic diet on glycemic control in diabetic patients: meta-analysis of clinical trials. *Cureus*. 2020;12(10):e10796.

Bueno NB, de Melo IS, de Oliveira SL, et al. Very-low-carbohydrate ketogenic diet v. low-fat diet for long-term weight loss: a meta-analysis of randomised controlled trials. *British Journal of Nutrition*. 2013;110(7):1178–87.

Ciaffi J, Mitselman D, Mancarella L, et al. The effect of ketogenic diet on inflammatory arthritis and cardiovascular health in rheumatic conditions: a mini review. *Frontiers in Medicine (Lausanne)*. 2021;8:792846.

Coffey D. "Does the human body replace itself every 7 years?" *Life's Little Mysteries*. Life Science. 2022. https://www.livescience.com/33179-does-human-body-replace-cells-seven-years.html.

Davis JJ, Fournakis N, Ellison J. Ketogenic diet for the treatment and prevention of dementia: a review. *Journal of Geriatric Psychiatry and Neurology*. 2021; 34(1):3–10.

Di Raimondo D, Buscemi S, Musiari G, et al. Ketogenic diet, physical activity, and hypertension–a narrative review. *Nutrients*. 2021;13(8):2567.

Drabińska N, Wiczkowski W, Piskuła MK. Recent advances in the application of a ketogenic diet for obesity management. *Trends in Food Science & Technology*. 2021;110:28–8.

Haslam RL, Bezzina A, Herbert J, et al. Can ketogenic diet therapy improve migraine frequency, severity and duration? *Healthcare (Basel)*. 2021;9(9):1105.

Heinke P, Rost F, Rode J, et al. Diplod hepatocytes drive physiological liver renewal in adult humans. *Cell Systems*. 2022;13:499–507.

Kong G, Wang J, Li R, et al. Ketogenic diet ameliorates inflammation by inhibiting the NLRP3 inflammasome in osteoarthritis. *Arthritis Research & Therapy*. 2022;24(1):113.

Luong TV, Abild CB, Bangshaab M, et al. Ketogenic diet and cardiac substrate metabolism. *Nutrients*. 2022;14:1322.

Mundi MS, Mohamed Elfadil O, Patel I, et al. Ketogenic diet and cancer: fad or fabulous? *JPEN: Journal of Parenteral & Enteral Nutrition*. 2021;45(S2):26–32.

Pavón S, Lázaro E, Martínez O, et al. Ketogenic diet and cognition in neurological diseases: a systematic review. *Nutrition Review*. 2021;79(7):802–13.

Phillips MCL, Murtagh DKJ, Gilbertson LJ, et al. Low-fat versus ketogenic diet in Parkinson's disease: a pilot randomized controlled trial. *Movement Disorders*. 2018;33(8):1306–14.

Sampaio LP. Ketogenic diet for epilepsy treatment. *Arq Neuropsiquiatr*. 2016;74(10):842–8.

Saslow LR, Mason AE, Kim S, et al. An online intervention comparing a very low-carbohydrate ketogenic diet and lifestyle recommendations versus a Plate Method Diet in overweight individuals with type 2 diabetes: a randomized controlled trial. *Journal of Medical Internet Research*. 2017;19(2):e36.

Shimazu T, Hirschey MD, Newman J, et al. Suppression of oxidative stress by þ-hydroxybutyrate, an endogenous histone deacetylase inhibitor. *Science*. 2013;399(6116):211–4.

Snopek L, Mlcek J, Sochorova L, et al. Contribution of red wine consumption to human health protection. *Molecules*. 2018;23(7):1684.

Spalding KL, Bergmann O, Alkass K, et al. Dynamics of hippocampal neurogenesis in adult humans. *Cell*. 2013;153(6):1219–27.

Stiepan D. "Mayo Clinic Minute: Relationship between food, disease stronger than you may think." Mayo Clinic. 2022. https://newsnetwork.mayoclinic.org/discussion/mayo-clinic-minute-mayo-clinic-minute-relationship-between-food-disease-stronger-than-you-may-think.

Talib WH, Mahmod AI, Kamal A, et al. Ketogenic diet in cancer prevention and therapy: molecular targets and therapeutic opportunities. *Current Issues in Molecular Biology*. 2021;43(2):558–89.

Weber DD, Aminzadeh-Gohari S, Tulipan J, et al. Ketogenic diet in the treatment of cancer – Where do we stand? *Molecular Metabolism*. 2020;33:102–21.

Whalen C, Mattie F, Bach E, et al. A ketogenic diet is protective against atherosclerosis in apolipoprotein E knockout mice. *Current Developments in Nutrition*. 2020;4(Suppl 2):87.

Wheless JW. History of the ketogenic diet. *Epilepsia*. 2008;49(S8):3–5.

Włodarczyk A, Cubała WJ, Stawicki M. Ketogenic diet for depression: a potential dietary regimen to maintain euthymia? *Progress in Neuro-Psychopharmacology and Biological Psychiatry.* 2021;109:110257.

Włodarczyk A, Cubała WJ, Wielewicka A. Ketogenic diet: a dietary modification as an anxiolytic approach? *Nutrients.* 2020;12(12):3822.

Zhu H, Bi D, Zhang Y, *et al.* Ketogenic diet for human diseases: the underlying mechanisms and potential for clinical implementations. *Signal Transduction and Targeted Therapy.* 2022;7:11.

■ CHAPTER 11

Bitok E, Sabaté J. Nuts and cardiovascular disease. *Progress in Cardiovascular Diseases.* 2018;61(1):33–7.

Bauset C, Martínez-Aspas A, Smith-Ballester S, et al. Nuts and metabolic syndrome: reducing the burden of metabolic syndrome in menopause. *Nutrients.* 2022;14(8):1677.

Casas-Agustench P, Bulló M, Salas-Salvadó J. Nuts, inflammation and insulin resistance. *Asia Pacific Journal of Clinical Nutrition.* 2010;19(1):124–30.

Kerimi A, Williamson G. The cardiovascular benefits of dark chocolate. *Vascular Pharmacology.* 2015;71:11–5.

Ros E, Singh A, O'Keefe JH. Nuts: natural pleiotropic nutraceuticals. *Nutrients.* 2021;13(9):3269.

Rul F, Béra-Maillet C, Champomier-Vergès MC, et al. Underlying evidence for the health benefits of fermented foods in humans. *Food & Function.* 2022;13(9):4804–24.

Thomas L. "Resveratrol in Wines and Grapes." News Medical. 2021. https://www.news-medical.net/health/Resveratrol-in-Wines-and-Grapes.aspx.

Index